LES
MORE LIFE

FIND OUT WHY YOUR BEST EFFORTS AREN'T WORKING

ANSWERS TO THE TOP 21 WEIGHT LOSS QUESTIONS

LESS WAIST MORE LIFE

FIND OUT WHY YOUR BEST EFFORTS AREN'T WORKING

ANSWERS TO THE TOP 21 WEIGHT LOSS QUESTIONS

Thomas W. Clark, MS, MD, FACS

Board Certified Bariatric Surgeon and Bariatrician

Center for Weight Loss Success, PC

LESS WAIST MORE LIFE

FIND OUT WHY YOUR BEST EFFORTS
AREN'T WORKING

ANSWERS TO THE TOP 21
WEIGHT LOSS QUESTIONS

© 2013 Thomas W. Clark, MS, MD, FACS

Published by Adriel Publishing

Edited by Karol H. Clark, MSN, RN

FIRST EDITION

Printed in the U.S.A.

Cover design by Liz Lawless

ISBN-13: 978-1-939998-03-3

www.cfwls.com

Dedication

I dedicate this book to anyone who struggles with their weight and wants to end their frustrating weight loss roller coaster ride. I commend you for your commitment to not only lose weight, but understand how to keep it off for life. I am honored to be a part of your journey.

I also dedicate this book to the passionate staff of professionals at CFWLS who are committed to helping our patients learn what they "can" do, rather than what they "can't" do in order to lose weight and live the life they desire and deserve.

Finally, I dedicate this book to my wife of 21 years and our children – Kendall, Daniel, Mason & Kaylen who make us smile and help to keep us young!

Disclaimer

Some of the information in this book is anecdotal opinions from the author after practicing extensively and exclusively in the field of bariatric surgery (performing nearly 4,000 primary weight loss surgery procedures) and bariatric medicine. Unless otherwise stated, statements are based upon his extensive clinical experience (and common sense) over the past 20 years specializing in bariatric surgery and bariatric medicine.

The testimonials are from actual clients of Dr. Clark and the Center for Weight Loss Success. The opinions of these clients are theirs and freely given.

The individuals described in each chapter reflecting upon the question at hand are based on actual clients and their personal situations. However, the name identified within the chapter has been changed for their privacy.

The information presented in this book is guidelines set forth by the author for his patients. This information is individualized for them by the author and the professional staff at the Center for Weight Loss Success based upon their particular situation.

Individual medical advice must be modified based upon the patient's individual situation by his/her chosen bariatric physician and primary care practitioner. The information in this book is intended to serve as a guide to people who want to successfully lose weight and experience long-term results.

The information presented in this book is in no way intended to replace or contradict any and all information or physician orders set forth by your chosen bariatric surgeon, bariatric physician or primary care practitioner. All weight loss patients should seek specific advice and recommendations pertinent to their particular situation from their chosen bariatric surgeon/physician and primary care practitioner. Please contact your bariatric surgeon/physician and/or primary care practitioner with any specific medical/surgical questions you may have.

Table of Contents

A Note from the Author

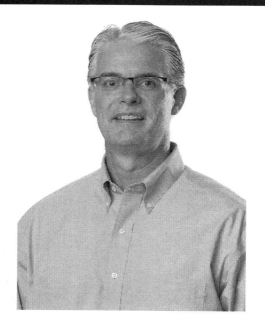

Thomas W. Clark, MS, MD, FACS

I love helping people lose weight! It's true! I also strive to be an example of how to integrate the strategies I share into your life … and actually *enjoy* it!

I follow the strategies set forth in this book, but that hasn't always been the case. Morbid obesity runs in my family and if I am not careful, I have the propensity to gain weight very easily. About four years ago, my wife and I participated in our *Dr. Clark's Jump Start Diet.* It is a 2 week nutritionally sound program intended to jump start your weight loss and give you the motivation to continue to improve your health. I couldn't believe it – I lost 23 pounds and gained the energy to begin a rigorous exercise program. My wife lost 11 pounds and did the same. To tell you the truth, I haven't looked back and have kept the weight off ever since. I have also significantly improved my lean body mass. For those times I *choose* to indulge, I no longer have to beat myself up. I enjoy my chosen indulgence and then get back to what I know is best – and more importantly, what makes me feel my best so I can function at a much higher level. I only wish I had done it sooner.

You will hear stories from others throughout this book as well. Everyone's story is unique whether it is a weight loss of 5 pounds or 150+ pounds. We each made a conscious decision to take control of our life and lose weight. More than that, we chose to understand how to keep it off for life and take the necessary steps to do just that. My job is to help you do the same. My job is to try to take some of the guess work out of it so you can make the most of your weight loss efforts and see results that can last a lifetime. Your story may begin with what you think is a short-term "diet" but if you can turn that into a lifestyle you love – that's where the real long-term benefits and "ease" take over.

You are in luck! I love doing research – discovering the

"why" behind what works and what doesn't intrigues me. I not only diligently review the "best of the best", I also integrate these strategies for weight loss and fitness into my life. I also break it down into simple to understand tips and share this information with you on a weekly basis via easy (usually free) tools. These tools include podcasts, articles for local publications, webinars, social media, national public presentations, activities and events. At CFWLS, I surround myself with licensed/certified professionals who share my passion and have the gift of helping others integrate these behaviors and this knowledge into their lives and their particular situations.

I've done the tedious work so you don't have to. In this book, I simplify the latest research and share answers to the top 21 questions my staff and I are asked nearly every day. You will likely identify with many of the people you will meet. I will share with you what I know ... about what works and what doesn't. Why some current beliefs can actually prevent you from losing weight and how to efficiently make the most of your weight loss efforts. I am your biggest fan and I want you to be successful. Helping people lose weight and understand how to keep it off is my mission in life. This gives meaning to what I do every day.

About the Author

Dr. Clark is a highly sought after board certified bariatric surgeon and bariatrician. Dr. Clark has performed nearly 4,000 weight loss surgery procedures, making him one of the most experienced bariatric surgeons in the world. He is uniquely able to help people who have struggled with their weight finally attain long-term weight loss success with his exclusive Weight Management University™ programs. Dr. Clark has been a hospital Bariatric Program Medical Director for over 10 years. He is a frequent speaker at the American Society of Bariatric Physicians, presents research at the American Society for Metabolic and Bariatric Surgery, and participates in other national conferences. Dr. Clark is a best-selling author of the 'More Life' book series and founder of the Center for Weight Loss Success in Newport News, VA. This center is a state-of-the-art facility for medial weight loss, surgical weight loss, fitness and nutrition. Learn more about Dr. Clark, his professional staff and his comprehensive center of excellence at www.cfwls.com.

Foreword

KENNY'S STORY

A ROCKING INSPIRATION!

I've been a drummer in a rock band almost my entire life. Thinking back to before I joined the program I had hip issues due to being heavier than I had ever been. I have small children and I want to be around awhile longer for them. Dropping some weight and improving my health was necessary. I absolutely hated exercise but assumed it was the 'Nature of the Beast'! I decided that I was going to dig in and take 3 months to make this happen. I participated in the program with a good friend and co-worker to help push me a bit and lend support as well as add a bit of competition.

My habits at work were working against me. In the morning, I would just grab something and then later get a bag of chips from the machine. I would have some crackers in the afternoon and then later grab a cupcake and knew that was the kind of thing that had to stop.

Weight Management University™ is an awesome program. It's off the charts awesome! I was really skeptical at first. Two weeks prior to the program starting, I was looking at a hip replacement because the pain was intolerable. Now it's still sore from time to time but it's something that I can live with. This program has turned my life around.

When I first met with a counselor and she asked what kind of activity I liked to do, I told her that biking was my thing. I have a Harley that I really love to ride, but she smiled and rephrased the question. How did I preferred burning calories? I use to hate exercise, but I've learned to actually enjoy it and it's become part of my regular routine. I feel good after I've worked out and I feel like I've accomplished something.

I set personal goals and to achieve these goals, I had to step it up a notch. I couldn't just continue to do the right things with my foods and eating healthier, I had to do something extra, that was where the exercise came in. I feel 100 times better. Before, by 4 o'clock in the afternoon, when I got off work, it was home to the couch. Now at 4 o'clock, I'm looking forward to 5:30 so that I can go work out! I can ride my bike (the kind with pedals!) with my kids. It's actually something I look forward to.

There were little mini-stories along the way. So many people could see my progress and wanted to know what I was doing to lose weight. I shared what I was learning every week in class to help others enjoy the same benefits that I was seeing. Having a buddy in the program was great because we pushed each other and never wanted to let the other down.

This isn't rocket science. I didn't get a shot in the arm. I was taught what to eat and how to look for what to eat and how to exercise. They made learning fun. The most intriguing part of the program was seeing how I could grow as a person. Having my goal weight out there was my carrot and sometimes that meant behaving a bit better on my weekends. It's a lifestyle change. It's watching what I eat and keeping track of it (Calories, Carbs & Protein). It's drinking water instead of sodas. I lost just over 45 pounds in 3 months and I did it with the help of Weight Management University™ and the staff at the Center for Weight Loss Success. Now when I am behind the drum set with the rest of my band I feel that I really can "Rock all night long"!

Before

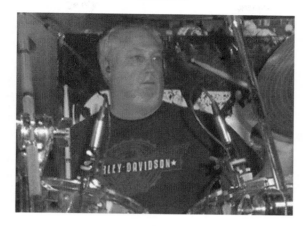

After

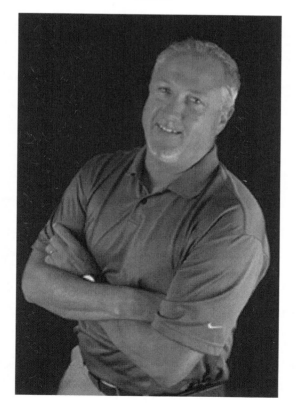

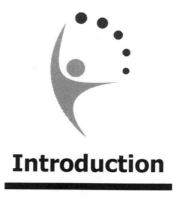

Introduction

At the time this book was written, the Centers for Disease Control & Prevention report that more than one-third of U.S. adults (35.7% or 97 million people) are obese1. You might want to read that sentence again. They also confirm that being obese increases your incidence of obesity-related conditions including heart disease, stroke, Type 2 diabetes and certain types of cancer. These obesity conditions are identified as the second leading cause of preventable death in the United States2.

The purpose of this book is not to create blame or focus on the negative. It's not entirely the fault of individuals such as you. You are bombarded with conflicting advice and information. On one hand this drives us to higher levels of research, but on the other hand, it creates communities of people who think they are practicing healthy behaviors when in fact, they are potentially sabotaging their best efforts to lose weight.

It is clearly time to take control of this dismal statistic and improve the health of our nation one person, one family, and one community at a time. You do not need to be another "preventable" statistic. We want you to free yourself from the disease called obesity and potentially influence others to do the same. Feeling your best provides you with the opportunity to perform better in your chosen career and experience a full life with those that you care about most. That's what life is all about!

This is why our mission at the Center for Weight Loss Success (CFWLS) is *to create a community of motivated people who understand how to manage their weight for life.* It's also why we created Losing Weight USA (www.losingweightusa.com) and provide individual coaching so you can integrate healthy behaviors within the constraints of your unique environment. It's not enough to provide quality education. For successful change, you must *want* to change (motivation) and believe you have the ability to change. Daily behaviors and habits must be modified.

It is more than willpower. Reading this book won't make you change (only you can decide to make that happen) but it is a start in the right direction and will provide you with the necessary tools to effectively begin your journey and take action to a healthier you. We see success each and every day and you can too!

In nearly all circumstances, it is believed that informed decisions generally make for better decisions. Informed decisions require some degree of research and education. Thus, if you are seeking successful weight loss, it's a good idea to do your homework so that this time it isn't just "one more diet that didn't work". This book will help you with your homework since it answers the most common weight loss questions you may wonder about along with the answers to questions you may not have thought to ask.

Long-term weight loss is much more than just a "diet". It is a wonderful and rewarding way of life that is well within your reach. This is especially true if you can honestly answer "Yes" to the following two questions after reading this book:

1. Can I do this?

2. Is it worth it?

If you can answer yes to these two questions after reading this book, success can be yours. You will be more likely to follow the recommendations set forth in this book and understand why such positive changes are important to you (which keeps you on the right track). These answers will help you on your journey to health and also introduce you to a bigger step-by-step plan that will change your life and simplify weight loss so you don't have to imagine your life without the difficulties of being overweight. You can actually experience how it feels – sooner than you think!

Thank you for purchasing this book. As an added bonus, you can visit the website www.weightlosssuccess4me.com and log in to download 21 free videos I personally created that accompany this book along with two additional free reports "Why can't I lose weight? and "9 Ways to Jump Start Your Weight Loss". I can't wait to hear about your successful weight loss journey. Our main website is also full of free resources such as free podcasts, blogs, social media links and more to help you lose weight. Visit often at www.cfwls.com. If you are interested in weekly access to me for a "how to" webinar, weekly tip sheets, recipes and more, you will want to join Losing Weight USA at www.LosingWeightUSA.com. Remember ... It's your life ... make it a healthy one.

[1]http://www.cdc.gov/obesity/data/adult.html

[2]http://www.nhlbi.nih.gov/guidelines/obesity/ob_gdlns. htm

CHAPTER 1

I EAT HEALTHY SO WHY AM I NOT LOSING WEIGHT?

*M*eet Kelly: *Kelly arrives at the Center for Weight Loss Success (CFWLS) smiling but obviously frustrated ... almost tearful. She is well groomed and soft spoken. She is prompt and obviously organized. Kelly is 39 and mother of two young girls. She is educated and grew up on a farm in Ohio where fruits and vegetables were abundant. She did not have a weight problem until after the birth of her children. Kelly is 25 pounds above her desired weight and fatigued. As she sits in the consultation office, she seems a bit uncomfortable ... almost embarassed that she is here at all.*

She wants to lose this weight and can't figure out why she is having trouble and feeling so tired. Especially since she follows the advice of her mother and many family magazines indicating she and her family should eat healthy by including plenty of fruits & vegetables, whole grains, and low fat food alternatives.

How many times have you heard it? "Eat plenty of fruits and whole grains for healthy eating" – and there is some truth to that. Fruits and whole grain foods have plenty of fiber, antioxidants, flavenoids and phytonutrients just to name a few. But … they also have significantly higher amounts of carbohydrate … which are *all* eventually broken down into *sugar*. This isn't a problem unless you are sensitive to carbohydrates (and almost everyone is to some extent). If that is the case, then eating plenty of fruits and whole grains will NOT help you lose weight. "Healthy Eating" and "Eating for Weight Loss" are NOT the same thing.

That does not mean that you can't eat healthy while you are eating to lose weight. It just means that there are certain foods which are considered "good for you" that you will need to keep to a very minumum while you are *eating to lose weight.*

Let me explain further as I share with you what "carbohydrate sensitivity" is and what you can do to control it. More importantly, what you can do to prevent your progression from carbohydrate sensitivity to insulin resistance and eventually Type 2 Diabetes.

You should know that if you are obese (Body Mass Index > 30), your risk of developing diabetes is considered 80% higher than someone at a normal weight. Once properly diagnosed, controlling your carbohydrate sensitivity can radically change how you feel (for the better) and positively impact your ability to lose weight.

Blood sugar, also known as glucose, is the primary source of energy or fuel for all of our body's cells. Your body makes glucose by breaking down carbohydrates and proteins to be utilized as fuel. You may not be aware, but fats do not break down into glucose. Rather, fats break down into ketones which can also be utilized as fuel.

The most desirable fasting blood sugar levels range from 70 to 100 with the optimal being in the low 80's. Fasting blood sugar, of course, is measured after not eating for about 8 to 12 hours. After you consume your meal, however, the food is digested and broken down. Proteins are broken down resulting in very slow rises – and sometimes decreases – in blood sugar. Carbohydrates are broken down into simple sugars (glucose) and cause a more rapid rise of blood sugar.

As your blood sugar rises, a signal is sent to your pancreas to secrete the hormone insulin. Insulin allows sugar to be taken into your cells and utilized as energy. Insulin is a necessary 'escort', so to speak. *Normally* your blood sugar can rise immediately after eating to approximately 120 but is regulated by insulin to bring your blood sugar levels down to that optimal 80's range.

Your body normally does a great job keeping things fairly regulated. But there is a condition called carbohydrate sensitivity or reactive hypoglycemia. This usually occurs after the consumption of a high carbohydrate meal (usually after life long, continuous high carbohydrate eating). There is a delay in the normal insulin release resulting in a blood sugar spike. This is followed by an over production of insulin, which then over supplies the blood stream and can drop your blood sugars to an unhealthy low level.

These blood sugar swings may produce the symptoms of:

- Fatigue
- Dizziness
- Irritability
- Inability to concentrate
- Shakiness
- Headaches

But these swings also initiate hunger and cravings, usually for more carbohydrates, which then starts the cycle over again. These low blood sugar levels are usually preceded by significant high blood sugars.

These swings can be evaluated by looking at some of your

lab values, particularly your hemoglobin A1C (HgA1C). In a simplified explanation, comparing, your HgA1C with your fasting blood sugar can determine how high a blood sugar swing you have had over the previous 3 months.

Adjusting your eating habits is the best way to minimize your carbohydrate sensitivity and significantly improve or eliminate the adverse symptoms identified above. Lowering your carbohydrate intake, particularly the simple sugars, will keep you from over-secreting the insulin and keep your blood sugar swings under control. Exercising also helps improve carbohydrate sensitivity.

As an additional note: When food labels of "low fat" alternatives are compared to regular options, you will generally notice an increase in the carbohydrate content. You will want to keep an eye out for this and avoid such options if you are diagnosed as being carbohydrate sensitive and trying to control your carbohydrate intake. Fat is what adds a great deal of flavor to food and helps to keep you satisfied. If it is removed, carbohydrate is commonly added to enhance the taste.

What can Kelly do? Kelly can work with an experienced physician to determine if she has carbohydrate sensitivity or any other underlying reason for her weight gain. In addition, reading food labels and eating the best lower carbohydrate food choices she enjoys will help her control her symptoms (such as her fatigue) and improve her ability to lose weight. Individualized counseling, education and integration of fitness (including weight training) will help her attain her weight loss goal. These skills/actions will also be a positive/healthy influence for her family.

Stephanie's Story

I am so happy to have reached my weight loss goals. I couldn't have done it without the help of the team members at Dr. Clark's Center for Weight Loss Success. The education and support I received not only helped me reach my goals, it is now helping me maintain my new and improved lifestyle. I have lost 47 pounds and I love it!

Before

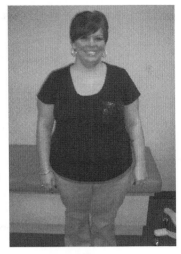

After

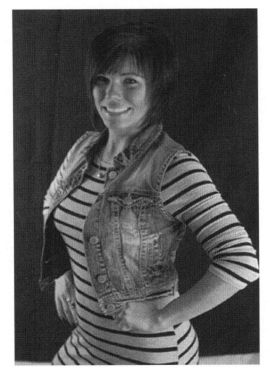

CHAPTER 2

IS THERE A "QUICK FIX" OR PILL
I CAN TAKE TO LOSE WEIGHT?

*M*eet Michael: *Michael can't even believe he has taken time out of his busy schedule to visit CFWLS. His wife has been nagging him to lose weight and made the appointment for him ... even drove him here because she knew otherwise he would find an excuse to not show up or re-schedule the appointment. He is obviously annoyed at his situation and the fact that he snores every night, has high blood pressure and has used work as an excuse to avoid family activities that involve physical exertion. He wants to lose weight. His primary care physician even told him he needs to* lose weight, but he doesn't have time to make it happen. It's tough taking the time while running an accounting firm. Yet, he wants to lose weight for himself, his family and for his overall presentation with clients. He wants a quick fix and these problems to go away as soon as possible with minimal or no effort.

Wouldn't it be great if there was a safe "pill" you could take to lose weight? If there was, then I would have a different career and you wouldn't likely be reading this book. There are some "quick fix" programs that provide short-term results and work quite well. Unfortunately, quick fix solutions generally do not address underlying problems that likely caused you to become overweight in the first place.

Let's take a look at what "quick fix" solutions may offer and how effective they may (or may not) be. At CFWLS, we do offer a "quick fix" plan for people such as Michael. The plan is outlined below and is nutritionally sound. If followed properly, you will experience an average weight loss of 5-25 pounds in 2 weeks, depending your gender (men tend to lose more weight – a separate discussion) and your level of activity or fitness.

At CFWLS, we currently offer two separate "quick plans". They include Dr. Clark's Jump Start Diet (all supplements for 2 weeks for those that want quick results with no food preparation or planning) and the "Quick Fix" plan. Both are described on our website at www.cfwls.com. However, I will go into further detail here on the Quick Fix plan since it incorporates food as well – which sometimes causes some confusion.

The CFWLS "Quick Fix" plan is a food and protein supplementation diet consisting of approximately 1,100-1,200 calories depending on food choices you select. It is ideal if you want to "accelerate" your weight loss and get on the right track with a flexible healthy eating plan. The afternoon snack may be taken mid-morning instead. Although this is developed as a 2 week "Quik Fix" plan, since it is so nutritionally complete, the plan may be continued longer. The shakes referenced are very filling since they contain casein protein (see Question 19) and are available at www.cfwls.com.

CFWLS *Quick Fix* 2 Week Plan

Breakfast: (200 calories): 1 Weight and Inches shake

Lunch: (200 calories): 1 Weight and Inches shake

*Afternoon Snack: (200 calories) 1 Weight and Inches shake

Main Meal: (approx. 500-600 calories): Include protein, salad, and vegetable.

Protein (approx.. 200-250 calories): 1 serving daily from the following with all skin, bone, visible fat removed and use a cooking method that does not add fat. Some choices include:

- 5 oz ground beef (lean 10%), very lean steak, veal or pork

- 6 oz chicken or turkey (white meat only)
- 6 oz venison or lean ham
- 6-8 oz white fish, shell fish, or canned fish (must be water packed or rinsed)

*If you prefer, you can have one of the CFWLS protein bars for an afternoon snack instead of the third Weight & Inches Shake. However, the bars (though convenient) have more calories and carbohydrates. As a result, I recommend using no more than 1 bar per day.

Salad (approx. 50 calories):

- 2 cups lettuce or other leafy greens
- 1 cup vegetables (celery, tomato, cucumber, etc.)

AND

- Low calorie dressing (25 calorie limit) OR vinegar, salt, lemon juice and other desire spices

Vegetables (approx. 50-100 calories):

- Choose 1 cup cooked broccoli, spinach, beets, asparagus, carrots, green beans or cauliflower

Water/Beverages: TRY TO DRINK at least 8 cups (64oz) of water each day.

You can drink other beverages as long as they are calorie-free (less than 5 calories per serving) and caffeine-free. Suggestions for these types of beverages include decaf coffee and tea, decaf diet soda, Crystal Light, diet seltzer or diet mineral water, and herbal teas. Remember, caffeine acts as a diuretic and causes you to lose water from your body. If you must have caffeine please limit to one serving per day.

Journaling: We recommend that all of our patients begin journaling your food and fluid intake as well as daily exercise. We will want you to continue journaling throughout your weight loss journey to help you become more conscious of your food selections and intake – and to track your success!

To get the most out of this plan, I also recommend these 4 additional vitamins/nutrients that are included in this diet (check with your experienced bariatric physician/surgeon):

- Complete Multi-Vitamin (2 tabs/day)
- Activated B-Complex (1-2 capsules/day)
- Magnesium/Potassium Aspartate (1 twice/day)
- Essential Fatty Acids (1-2 grams/day)

Another option you may be considering is a "fast". It may seem like the perfect solution to you for quick and easy weight loss. After all haven't spiritual leaders been doing it safely for years? And because weight loss fasting can be a test of willpower, won't it help us to develop discipline and confidence?

While fasting may be tempting for quick weight loss, it is actually not recommended for many reasons. First, it sets you up for failure due to feelings of deprivation (and usually a resulting binge). Second, your body reverts to "fight or flight" status and slows down your metabolism in preparation for scarcity of food. Your lean body mass is sacrificed which drives your overall metabolism down (more on this in Question 6). Thus, while you may experience short-term weight loss (primarily water loss), this is not a viable long-term plan.

What can Michael do? Michael can consider a Jump Start or Quick Fix plan which are both nutritionally sound and provides for adequate amounts of quality protein. Based upon his medical conditions, he would do himself a favor if he took the time to meet with an experienced bariatric physician, evaluated necessary laboratory tests and implemented a long-term weight loss plan that incorporates his likes/dislikes, needs and lifestyle. Plans such as this can be implemented in very convenient ways. For example, at CFWLS, we provide effective online options such as podcasts, webinars and Skype/Telephone coaching (although in person is always best). In addition, fitness can be accomplished in many convenient ways from workouts at home, fitness centers or personal training during a time chosen by the client. One cookie-cutter program doesn't generally work well for people such as Michael so he will want to make sure his plan is able to be customized.

CHAPTER 3

WHAT SHOULD I LOOK FOR IN A WEIGHT LOSS PROGRAM?

*M*eet Desiree: *Desiree has had a wake-up call. Her physician has indicated that unless she loses about 75 pounds, her diabetes will worsen requiring higher levels of insulin, her degenerative joint disease may result in her need to use a cane or wheelchair, she will need to go on a CPAP machine for her sleep apnea and she will soon require an additional anti-hypertensive medication to control her blood pressure. Desiree is scared. She wonders how it got to this. Desiree is frightened and tearful. She needs help but wants to make sure she makes the best choice that is effective and affordable for her.*

All weight loss programs are not the same. There are so many to choose from, it is downright confusing. Not only are there a lot of weight loss programs to choose from, there are just as many fitness and nutritional options. It's no wonder care is often fragmented resulting in less than optimal outcomes.

When determining what weight loss program is right for you, you may just want to ask the following initial burning questions:

- What programs/services do you offer?
- What does it cost?
- Will it work for me?

However, you would be doing yourself a favor if you also asked the following questions:

- Is your program implemented and/or supervised by a physician?
- Is your physician board certified?
- How much experience does your physician have?
- How long have you been in business?
- What is the staff credentials/experience?
- For bariatric physicians, ask – Are you a member of ASBP (American Society for Bariatric Physicians)? For bariatric surgeons, ask – Are you a member of ASMBS (American Society for Metabolic & Bariatric Surgery)?

- Based on my personal health and weight, what program/services do you recommend for me? Why?
- Do you recommend any laboratory tests? Which ones and why?
- What are your average outcomes?
- Do you offer comprehensive services including nutritional coaching, fitness, ongoing support groups, ongoing education and availability of a psychologist?
- Do you have a dietician or nutritionist available to patients?
- How are questions during non-office hours handled?
- Do you have patients who are willing to share their experiences with me?

Questions are one part of the equation and your level of comfort and/or trust is another. You will get a "feel" for the office/program/staff from your first visit to their website, initial phone call and the moment you walk through the door. Weight loss doesn't have to be uncomfortable or a drudgery. Select a program that you *want* to participate in and one where you feel welcome. One where your specific needs will be met. Choose a program that has an outstanding track record for success led by professionals trained specifically in the area of weight loss, nutrition and fitness.

Ideally, you will be able to find a center that offers expert physician supervision/interaction, nutritional coaching by licensed professionals, ongoing education, delicious nutritional products (yes I said delicious – after I approve the nutritional content of the products we offer, we taste test everything and let you do the same), fitness classes/personal training with certified professionals all in a motivating, non-judgmental and fun environment.

What can Desiree do? Desiree can begin her research by talking with her primary care physician regarding options in her area. Having 75 pounds to lose with other health problems, she may also consider weight loss surgery. She will want to select a physician that will work closely with her primary care physician because her medications will need to be adjusted as she loses significant amounts of weight – hopefully to the point of medication elimination! Desiree will want to keep these questions handy and use them as she seeks the program/professionals right for her. She will require comprehensive program that includes laboratory analysis, evaluation by a bariatrician, individualized coaching, ongoing education and fitness classes that are non-threatening and fun. To lose 75 pounds, her optimal medical weight loss program will need to last at least 6 months to one year.

John's Story

After my younger brother passed away, I felt like I needed to do something about my health. I talked with my Doctor and we discussed weight loss surgery. I did not feel like that was for me and he told me about Dr Clark's medical weight loss program.

I got in touch with Dr Clark's office and joined Weight Management University. This has been the best decision I ever made. I started the program in May 2012. I started out at 434 lbs. (not my highest weight) and a little over a year later I am 290 lbs.

WOW 144 lbs later and I am a different person, with more energy and able to do more things in life. Sounds like a fairytale but it was not that hard actually. I had so much support from Dawn whenever I had a question about food, workouts and supplements. If I had a question and was not scheduled for a appointment I could email her with a quick response. I was always greeted with a smile and a "Wow how much are you down now" from Ashley and Star when I came into the office. Kat and Tina were always very informative whenever I visited the store. Dr Clark's weekly webinars and website were very insightful and helpful. Best part is the webinars are archived on the website and available 24/7.

You WILL change your body if you listen and follow the program like it is outlined. The one thing I like the best is the onsite gym. I can go anytime during the day and up to 11 pm and be able to get my workouts in and not feel like I am surrounded by gym rats LOL. The gym is equipped with enough items to keep your workouts challenging but obtainable.

The program is incredible. It is packed with information, classes, webinars and a supportive staff to make the change effortless.

What has all this done for me? I had chronic back pain and I am now able to do lawn work in about an hour instead of 1/2 the day due to not having to take a break every 10 minutes to ease the pain. I sleep better, have more energy throughout the day, Blood pressure and cholesterol levels are now low normal. Overall I have a better quality of life now. I know I would not have been able to accomplish this without Weight Management University. I am looking forward to the next year and continued weight loss. Look for an update when I hit my goal weight of 220 lbs. :-)

Before

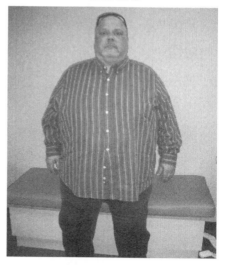

After

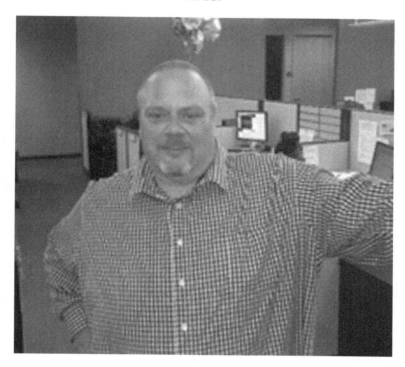

CHAPTER 4

Do I need to have any lab work or tests done before I begin?

*M*eet Carol: *Carol has three teenagers and leads an active life. She works full-time and has successfully sustained a healthy balance for work and home. Carol has always had to work at maintaining a healthy weight since morbid obesity runs in her family but has successfully done so all her life. She enjoys cooking when she can and exercising at least 3 times a week. Carol turned 50 two years ago. After that, everything began to change. She easily gained 5 pounds, then 10 pounds then 20 pounds and now 25 pounds causing a need for larger sizes since everything is too tight. Carol is frustrated and uncomfortable. She has increased* *her exercise and lowered her calorie intake but nothing seems to help. She is ready for a full "investigation" to find out what is going on.*

No matter what your situation, it is a good idea (and recommended) to obtain baseline values for certain laboratory tests in addition to completing a history and physical exam. Based upon recommendations from the American Society for Bariatric Physicians and my experience, the table below shows the laboratory tests most commonly ordered. You will also find the rationale for the test, normal results and what the significance is of the particular measurement. If you and your weight loss physician determine that an appetite suppressant may be utilized, a baseline EKG will be ordered as well.

LAB TEST	WHY PERFORMED	NORMAL VALUE	SIGNIFICANCE
TSH (Thyroid-Stimulating Hormone)	Screening test for abnormal thyroid function & used to evaluate thyroid hormone replacement	0.4-4.0 mIU/l	High levels may indicate hypothyroidism, thyroid hormone resistance. Low levels may indicate hyperthyroidism.
Cholesterol	To evaluate risks for heart disease.	Less than 200 mg/dL	The higher the level, the higher the risk for heart disease. High levels may be caused by diet, hypothyroidism, uncontrolled diabetes, liver problems or familial hyperlipidemias.
Triglycerides	Are compounds used by the body to move fatty acids through the blood.	Less than 150 mg/dL	High levels may put you at risk for heart disease even if your other lipid levels are within normal limits.
High Density Lipoprotein (HDL) Cholesterol	"Good or happy cholesterol" – takes excess cholesterol to the liver for excretion.	Equal or greater than 60 mg/dL	High levels will take away the increased risk from one risk factor and decrease your risk of heart disease. Levels below 40 mg/dL add a risk factor.

LAB TEST	WHY PERFORMED	NORMAL VALUE	SIGNIFICANCE
Hemoglobin	Is contained in RBC's & is the protein that carries oxygen in the blood.	May vary with altitude Male: 13.8-17.2 gm/dL Female: 12.1-15.1 gm/dL	Both high and low counts indicate defects with the balance of red blood cells in the blood and may indicate disease.
Hematocrit	Indicates the proportion of cells and fluids in the blood.	May vary with altitude. Male: 40.7-50.3% Female: 36.1-44.3%	Low values may indicate anemia, malnutrition. High levels may indicate dehydration.
Ferritin	A protein that stores iron in the body.	Male: 12-300 ng/ml Female: 12-150 ng/ml	The lower the ferritin, even within normal range, the more likely a patient is to be iron deficient. Low ferritin tends to stimulate certain cravings.
Vitamin B12	Helps in formation of RBC's and in the maintenance of the central nervous system.	211-911 PG/ml	Low levels can cause anemia as well as numbness or tingling in the extremities and other neurologic symptoms such as weakness and loss of balance.
Vitamin D	Fat soluble vitamin that helps the body absorb calcium for the normal mineralization of bone. Also called the "Sunshine Vitamin"	32-100 ng/mL	Low levels have been associated with falls, fractures, cancers, immune dysfunction, cardiovascular disease and high blood pressure and weight gain.
Folate	Necessary for the production of RBC's, synthesis of DNA & protein. Also helps with tissue growth and cell function.	>5.38 mcg/L	Deficiency causes poor growth, graying hair, inflammation of tongue, mouth ulcers, and diarrhea.
Glucose	Used to diagnose or screen for diabetes and to monitor control in patients who have diabetes.	Up to 100 mg/dL-ideally it should be 75-85	100-126 mg/dL-impaired fasting glucose or pre-diabetes. Diabetes is typically diagnosed when fasting levels are 120 mg/dL or higher.

Hemoglobin A1C (HgbA1C)	Gives a good estimate of how well blood sugars are being managed over time.	5% or less	The higher the value, the higher the risk of developing diabetic complications such as retinopathy, neuropathy, heart disease or stroke.
Fasting Insulin	Insulin is the pancreatic hormone that regulates blood sugar by facilitating glucose uptake by tissues – especially fat and skeletal muscle. Also stimulates fat storage and fluid retention. This measurement gives information about the body's sensitivity to insulin.	5-20 mcU/ml when fasting

Levels ≥ 8 indicate insulin resistance and carbohydrate sensitivity | Abnormal levels may indicate DM, obesity. Obesity decreases the sensitivity of various tissues to insulin, which normally results in the pancreas overcompensating and making excess insulin. High insulin, even with normal blood sugar, is caused by the body being resistant to insulin's effect – a condition called "insulin resistance syndrome" or "metabolic syndrome" which occurs commonly with obesity and polycystic ovary syndrome. |

Once you have your laboratory results, your weight loss physician will review them in detail with you. These results are very helpful in explaining underlying medical reasons why you may be having difficulty losing weight. All of this can be overwhelming, but your physician will be able to simplify it for you. When combined with your health history, physical exam, and review of your past efforts/symptoms/goals, your expert physician can determine the best weight loss plan for your particular situation.

What can Carol do? Carol is doing what she has always done … and what has always worked for her in the past. However, based upon the aging/menopausal process, these efforts are not effective for her any longer. That doesn't mean that she won't be able to lose her weight, it just means that it's not quite as simple as calories in/calories out. Carol needs to understand her current laboratory results and how her hormones may be affecting her ability to lose weight. She will also need to make some shifts in her workout routine to support weight loss and long-term success. Menopause is a complex subject so Carol will want to seek a physician who is experienced with not only weight loss but how such hormonal changes affects the ability to lose weight and how to maximize her efforts not only now but as she continues to age. With proper management, Carol can likely improve her health and potentially reverse some of the effects of aging on her body!

CHAPTER 5

How much weight can I expect to lose?

Meet Annette: Annette is vivacious, funny and beautiful. Her energy is infectious and she is all about the numbers. Her daughter is getting married in 6 months and her future mother-in-law is a size 8 and always looks great! Although Annette is confident and happy, she wants to look and feel her best (and secretly ... better than her daughter's future mother-in-law). She wants to lose 40 pounds by the date of the wedding. Annette completes her consultation and eagerly says "How much weight will I lose? Do you think I will lose 40 pounds in 6 months?"

The short answer for Annette is "yes". For medical weight loss, the average weight loss is 1-2 pounds per week. Thus, in six months there is a minimum of 24 weeks so that is an average weight loss of 24-48 pounds. At CFWLS, we see success every day. That success is experienced by individuals who have answered "yes" to the questions I discussed in the Introduction of this book – "Can I do this?" And "Is it worth it?" That indicates confidence and motivation. More than that, you need to commit to behavioral changes with regards to eating, fitness and follow-through with expert coaching advice.

Don't worry. This doesn't mean you are doomed to a life of sacrifice and drudgery. It is a lease on a new life and Annette (just like you) deserves to feel (and look) her very best. Each day you put off starting your weight loss plan is another day you choose to keep yourself from attaining your goal(s). Change is hard and often scary but this change is entirely worth it – you are going to have to trust me on this one!

There are a number of things that can and will affect your ability to lose the average amount of weight. I could write an entire chapter or book on many of these medical problems that can potentially adversely affect your ability to lose weight. However, a brief summary is listed below. If any of these affect you (or you think they may affect you), please discuss them in detail with your physician.

Diabetes:

- **Type II** diabetes is the end result of 6 to 15 years of insulin resistance with which your body has been dealing. Due to this insulin resistance, your pancreas cannot produce enough of the insulin your body needs to metabolize glucose. Your cells are hungry for energy but cannot get it without the help of oral medications or injections that give you the insulin you need. Your weight loss is dependent on the correct balance of diet with medication. There is also another type of diabetes that is unrelated to a history of poor eating habits or obesity known as Type I diabetes.

- **Type I** diabetes is the result of the pancreas islet cells (the actual cells that produce the insulin) dying off. The cause of Type I diabetes has been suspected as an autoimmune dysfunction as well as a possible viral exposure that initiated the autoimmune malfunction. With little to no insulin being produced, the body not only loses its fat storage abilities but it also must utilize what fat is already stored as its energy source. This is why unexplained weight loss may be the first symptom.

Adrenal Disorders:

The adrenal glands play a major role in day to day activities, releasing the "stress hormones" as we need them. One of these hormones called cortisol is a major player and when cortisol is released in higher than normal doses can lead to body changes that may be overlooked. Weight gain, particularly in the abdominal and back area, as well as the face (moon face) is just an outward symptom. High blood pressure, insulin resistance, high cholesterol and high triglycerides may also accompany this disease. A thorough examination and a few tests from your Primary Care Provider can determine a diagnosis of any of the adrenal gland disorders.

Puberty, Pregnancy, Menopause:

Some women may gain weight at times in their lives when there is a shift in their hormones - at puberty, during pregnancy, and at menopause. This is due to the changes in your female hormones, estrogen and progesterone. Estradiol, the primary estrogen produced by your ovaries, helps lower insulin levels as well as blood pressure. It also keeps your LDL levels low and your HDL levels high.

As women proceed through menopause your estradiol levels decrease taking away your natural ability to keep the abdominal weight off, the LDL levels increase and your HDL levels decrease. Magnifying the situation is the estrogen known as estrone, released by your adrenal glands as well as your fat cells. Estrone makes it easier to store fat. This hormone increases as your estradiol levels decrease, increasing your fat stores and therefore making more estrone and the fight becomes a continuous cycle.

Depression:

Many people who are depressed turn to eating to ease their emotional distress. Feeling hopeless and depressed can be an important reason for someone's difficulties with managing their weight. Eating healthy and exercising is essential to maintaining a healthy weight, but it is difficult to initiate these things when you are depressed.

Weight gain is a common result of depression. You might ask yourself when you began gaining the weight, or when you stopped enjoying exercise. The weight gain probably coincides with an emotional event, or a raised level of stress.

For many people eating can become both a source of comfort and frustration. It is a way in which you might respond to stress, and a way in which you might literally feed your low sense of self-esteem. It can become a vicious cycle in which you feel self-conscious because you are overweight and in turn respond to this feeling by overeating, or by avoiding exercise.

If you are having difficulty managing your weight as a result of depression, you should be aware that many antidepressants lead to weight gain on their own. This is no reason to avoid antidepressants, but it is also one of many good reasons not to use them for weight management. Increased levels of activity and exercise, in combination with an effort to eat well, will have an effect on your weight as well as your sense of self-confidence, control, and general well-being.

Hypothyroidism:

An underactive thyroid can bring your metabolism to a screeching halt causing unexplained and somewhat rapid weight gain. This also lowers your energy level and decreases your mental alertness. These symptoms can be confused with high blood sugar levels so it's always smart to have your thyroid hormones checked. There is a higher incidence in women as they get older (one in five).

The most common screening test for a low functioning thyroid is the TSH (Thyroid Stimulating Hormone). If your thyroid is determined to be the cause of your weight gain, following your physician's advice and taking your prescribed thyroid medication will regulate this problem and weight loss will be achievable.

Hyperthyroidism:

You would think that an over active thyroid would be a dream come true for weight management; however, increasing your metabolism is not the only effect it has on your body.

You will experience an uncomfortable rapid heart rate, become easily fatigued, have extreme hunger, feel excessively warm and feel nervous, anxious or irritable.

Hyperthyroidism may be accompanied by increased diarrhea, sweating and insomnia. Heart palpitations and arrhythmias are not unusual. Doesn't sound like a great way to lose weight ... does it?

Polycystic Ovarian Syndrome (PCOS):

Polycystic Ovarian Syndrome is one of the most common causes of infertility and menstrual irregularity. It may be recognized by three key diagnostic criteria: multiple ovarian cysts, excessive testosterone and elevated levels of insulin. Battling the insulin resistance by lowering your refined carbohydrate intake can help restore regular menses and fertility as well as help lose the abdominal weight associated with this syndrome.

Sleep Apnea or Other Sleep Disorders:

There is a strong correlation between weight and your inability to sleep well. Is it the weight that interferes with the sleep or is the lack of sleep causing the weight gain? Researchers have found that people who slept less than six hours or more than nine hours were more likely to have glucose tolerance problems leading to potential weight problems.

Researchers have also found that overweight people slept almost two hours less each week than did those of normal weight. Studies indicate that the less sleep women had, the more likely they were to gain weight. They have attributed this lack of sleep with an increase level of cortisol (the stress hormone) in addition to lower leptin levels and increased ghrelin levels, both appetite controlling hormones. This increased cortisol level seems to go hand in hand with an increase in insulin levels.

In addition to these medical conditions, there are numerous other conditions that may affect an individual's weight loss. Joint issues like arthritis may decrease your activity level. Chronic fatigue syndrome or fibromyalgia may also affect your desire to become more active, all of which will slow your weight loss progress.

Medications That Affect Weight Loss:

Due to the increase use of pharmaceuticals in treatment of the many disorders and diseases, medications have been added as a determinant of weight gain. There are certain categories of medications that are known for their side effect of weight gain.

Since **hormones** have an important role in your weight gain, those medications that regulate, influence or manipulate your hormone levels will affect your weight. Contraceptives, hormone replacement therapy (HRT) and infertility drugs, estrogen and progesterone products all affect the female's hormone levels.

Many **oral anti-diabetic** medications stimulate an increase in insulin secretion from your pancreas inducing the side effect of weight gain. Balancing your diet will greatly reduce your need for these medications.

Some of the best known weight-gainers include the **antipsychotic medications** as well as **some antidepressants.** The importance of the use of these medications may outweigh the concern over your weight.

Beyond medical issues, you are a product of your environment. Your emotions control to a great degree your behavior and how you respond to various situations as well. Thus, for most people, you go through life knowing what you have always known (or have been taught) and doing what you have always done. Then one day you wake up and realize that you are dissatisfied, unfulfilled, unhappy or maybe just scared. You hope that it's not too late. You realize that you should make some changes but you feel it is easier and more comfortable to continue knowing what you know and doing what you do. You try (may even succeed at positive changes) and then regress to the same old comfort zone. This results in continuation of the status quo and possibly a worsening of your situation.

You tell yourself you will start "do-ing" as soon as it is convenient ... next week ... next month ... after the hurricane ... after the summer/holiday is over ... you know the drill.

It's a cycle and many of you may be caught up in it ... frustrated ... maybe even knowing what to do ... but not doing it ... thinking you "should be more active" ... you "should eat healthier" ... you "should lose weight and get in shape". You may even "should" for others who think you "should eat everything on your plate", you "should eat junk food because you've had a rough day", and/or you "should not exercise because others need you more".

"Should-ing" comes in two forms. First, doing what you think others expect you "should" do despite what your hopes, conscience and gut are telling you to do. You feel guilty and want to feel approval from others so you give in. Second, is "should-ing" yourself by saying you "should" do something but not doing it because your conditioned over the years to behave otherwise. *Unfortunately "should-ing" doesn't make a difference. Do-ing does.*

For anyone like Annette, realizing the problem is an important first step. You must break the cycle of - You think → You want →You decide → You try → You fail (or temporarily succeed) You repeat. This is no way to live. You deserve better.

With regard to weight loss, this is particularly important if you are overweight (BMI between 25 and 29.9), obese (BMI

> 30), have high cholesterol, diabetes, high blood pressure, abnormal triglycerides, sleep apnea, are physically inactive and/or have a family history of heart disease (or just want to look/feel better). It's time to start "do-ing" ... NOW! Easier said than done ... I know and unfortunately, no one can do it for you. You need to take responsibility for losing weight and make it happen. It's never too late.

What can Annette do? Annette is motivated and ready. Annette needs to commit to a comprehensive program and lose 40 pounds. This is well within her reach! Annette will want to work with a team of experts so she can have a comprehensive work-up to determine if there are any underlying medical problems that need addressed. Then, an individualized plan can be implemented that fits into her schedule and lifestyle. She can focus on what she "can" do rather than what she "can't" do. Her eating plan will be key and she will need to incorporate resistance training/fitness in order to ensure that she maintains or increases her lean body mass throughout. Then she will be set-up for long-term success and a wedding day for her daughter that she can fully enjoy!

Linda's Story

I was diagnosed with diabetes. I could barely walk a few steps across the room without my knees hurting. I always had a cane. I could hardly get my breath, partially because of my diabetes but also because I was so out of condition. I was pretty much housebound. I had to have my husband with me when I went out of the house for assistance. It was very tough, it was lonely. I felt isolated.

I intended to have surgery, but my insurance wouldn't cover surgery until I had six months of nutritional counseling. During that six months as I was trying to follow the nutritional advice of my counselor, I began to lose weight on my own. So I decided to see if I could continue to lose weight that way.

I joined the medical weight loss program and I was really successful. It was the counseling every two weeks that really made the difference. It really answered any questions that I had. I was provided with educational reading material with questions that helped me apply the steps to my own life at home which really, really made me apply that to how I was living.

The exercise programs were also there and I felt that I couldn't participate in them at first but I soon realized that I could start at my own level. Now I just love it! You couldn't ask for a better bunch of people anywhere. I've worked all my life and I've never been anywhere that there were so many people that were so nice, so considerate, and so competent. I just love these people.

I can walk without a cane which I haven't done in years and it's just getting better all of the time. I have a lot more energy and my mood, my happiness is just off the charts. I was pretty depressed before, to be honest. Just do it. I would encourage you every way I can. Go to the next seminar or book a consultation with one of the staff at the Center for Weight Loss Success.

Before

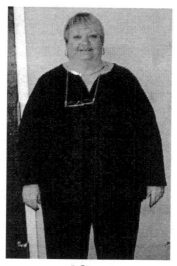

After

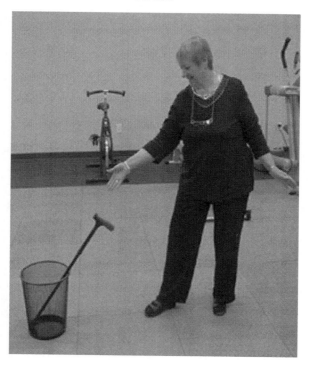

CHAPTER 6

What's my body composition and why should I care?

*M*eet Kate: *Kate is a nurse who has been struggling with her weight her entire life. She intellectually knows what to do but has a hard time with consistent implementation. She has always monitored her weight and clothing size but never really considered or understood why she would need to monitor any other information. Kate's weight has fluctuated up and down for as long as she can remember. Thus, much to her dismay, she keeps more than one size in her closet.*

Many people are only concerned with what they weigh. But what is at least as important is the **composition** of your weight. Meaning – how much is fat free mass/lean body mass (mainly muscle mass) and how much is fatty tissue.

The Lean Body Mass (LBM) is the healthy tissue. The fatty tissue is the unhealthy tissue. You want to get rid of your fatty tissue and keep (or even improve) your LBM. The more LBM you have, the higher your metabolism. If you are losing weight (good) but also losing LBM (muscle mass), what you are really doing is <u>slowing</u> your metabolism. When this happens, it will become harder for you to keep losing weight <u>and</u> easier to regain weight. So … it is imperative that you work to keep your LBM while you are losing weight and why we recommend you check your Body Composition on a regular basis throughout your weight loss process and beyond.

What do the numbers on a typical body composition analysis report mean?

The first number on your body composition analysis (BCA) is usually your weight – measured in pounds. This obviously is an important number since it is easy to measure. Just about everyone has a scale at home to check this. You should routinely weigh yourself since this is the measure of overall health easy to track.

The next number usually listed is your body fat. It is measured 2 ways: the percentage of fat that makes up your total weight (% body fat) and how many pounds of fat. During weight loss, you want to lose fat (see this number go down) NOT muscle.

After your body fat percentage, you will usually find your "Fat Free Mass" (FFM) identified. FFM is another way of saying Lean Body Mass (LBM – mainly your muscle). It is also measured 2 ways. These include the percentage of LBM that makes up your total weight (%FFM) and how many pounds of FFM you have.

During any weight loss plan, your LBM may be the most important number to track. It is your LBM that has a direct effect on your body's overall metabolism. It is extremely important to **preserve LBM** during your weight loss plan to **preserve your metabolism** (muscle burns more calories than fat).

You will likely also find your **total body water** on your BCA report. This gives you an idea of your overall hydration status and is also based on how much LBM you have. Your **Body Mass Index** is also calculated and found on your BCA report. This number is based on your height and weight. Anything over 30 is considered obese.

On many reports, you will often find an estimate of your **Resting Energy Expenditure (REE).** This is based on your gender, age, height and weight. It gives a close **approximation** of your basal metabolism. You generally need to take in about 500 calories less than this to see good weight loss (but I do not recommend going below 1000 calories/day). Your true basal metabolism can be measured, but it requires much more complex (and costly) testing to determine. Your "true" basal metabolism is based directly on how much muscle mass you have (the more the better). A pound of muscle burns approximately 50% more calories per day than a pound of fat.

Overall, keeping track of your body composition is important during weight loss. Especially keep track of your Lean Body Mass (LBM). You DO NOT want this number to go down since this means that your metabolism is slowing down. The best way to preserve LBM is the combination of taking in plenty of quality protein and exercise. Your weight loss physician can assist you with your particular macronutrient requirements (protein, carbohydrate and fat) along with your overall calorie requirement. Keep in mind that ongoing evaluation is necessary since as you get closer to your goal weight, you will need to determine your long-term macronutrient requirements, caloric recommendation and your carbohydrate ceiling (the maximum number of carbohydrates you can ingest without gaining weight). These numbers are different for everyone but significantly affects long-term weight loss success.

What should Kate do? Kate is armed with new knowledge and needs to put it to work for her. She likes tracking numbers and needs to get on a plan that she can live with while monitoring at least her weight, lean body mass and fat percentage. As she loses weight, she will want to make sure her lean body mass is at least the same or preferably increasing and her fat percentage decreasing. If she reaches her goal with this accomplished, her days of yo-yo dieting are more likely to be a thing of the past. Her metabolism will be able to support her new weight. If she works with her experienced physician/staff and can adopt a satisfying life of adequate protein, controlled carbohydrates and regular resistance training, she will experience the life many dream of and be a wonderful example for family and friends.

CHAPTER 7

HOW CAN I SPEED UP
MY WEIGHT LOSS?

*M*eet Mary Beth: *Mary Beth has wanted to lose weight for years. She is 45 years old and about 50 pounds overweight. Mary Beth has tried "everything" from diet plans and medications to exercise regimes and body cleanses. She has lost weight only to gain it back. She has a room full of exercise equipment at home and wants results now!!*

You may also want it now! You want that vision you have in your head of a slimmer, healthier you and you don't want it to take months or longer. Well … I would be lying if I said there was a way to get there without any effort, but there are ways to lose weight smarter … not harder. Here are some tips to get you there faster:

1. Stop counting calories and start counting carbs. The medical evidence is overwhelming that all carbohydrates break down into sugar which sets off a plethora of negative (fat storing) hormonal effects that will definitely keep you from success. If you are going to do just one thing, count your carbohydrate grams each day and try to initially keep them below 100 grams/day and then below 50 grams/day and you will be amazed! There is more to this than meets the eye. If you want to explore your individual carbohydrate "threshold", this will require additional effort and a consultation with your weight loss physician.

2. Stop making excuses and start making a plan. You are busy. It's a fact. However, you should not be too busy to take care of yourself and get your health in order and feel FANTAS-TIC. You are worth it. Take some time and think about what you really want to accomplish. Is it weight loss? Is it a particular size? Is it a lower blood pressure or blood sugar level? Is it decreasing joint pain? Is it feeling better about yourself? Is it all of the above? Figuring that out is the first step. Then break it down into baby steps so you don't get overwhelmed and throw in the towel. Once you know what you want to accomplish, begin setting a plan in place. There are many choices in terms of nutrition and fitness options to get you there but the most important thing is to do something ... something that will work for you. I'd like to say that just changing your eating or exercising more will do it but there must be a combination of dietary changes (you can live with for life), behavior changes (you can live with for life) and fitness (that you can live with for life). Whatever program you choose or whatever efforts you do on your own, make sure it includes all three.

3. Stop going, going, going and start doing, doing, doing. This gets back to your plan but there is more than that. It is effective execution of the plan and commitment to change. Getting your head in the game is half the battle. That will motivate you and then positive results (achieving your short-term goals) will keep you going.

4. Stop shopping for low fat and start shopping for low sugar. You will accomplish this by reading labels. Look at them. Anytime you find one that is "low fat" and you compare it to the regular alternative, you will find that the carbohydrate count is higher in the "low fat" one. Why? Because as I mentioned earlier, the flavor would be much worse and you wouldn't eat it. You will find the items with the highest carb/sugar content are located in the inner aisles of the grocery store. You are better off shopping around the periphery.

5. Eat twice as much protein each day as you do carbohydrates. We don't harp on weight loss in our family. We focus on eating when truly hungry, having an active life that includes family fitness and if my children ask about healthy eating, we discuss the simplest (yet very effective) advice (your protein/ carbohydrate ratio). Your first choice for eating should be lean protein (fish, chicken, eggs and cheese) then add colorful vegetables and salad.

6. Schedule fitness. You won't likely get it done unless it's on your schedule as a VERY important appointment.

These are general guidelines. You will need to have additional help if you have specific medical conditions or are considering surgical weight loss which requires a comprehensive program that includes education, coaching and fitness for optimal success.

Another consideration is your support system. If you want to lose weight, chances are you aren't the only one in your family or circle of friends who are trying to lose weight. You may think it is best to go it alone – it may be "safer" that way. You may believe that if you set your goals and keep them to yourself, you can protect yourself from a variety of risks such as criticism, exposure to public failure and needing to actually be "accountable" for your weight loss.

As I mentioned before, if everyone could do it on their own, we wouldn't likely have the weight problem in the world we do today. But there is a lot of confusing information "out there" and the reality is that change is usually uncomfortable.

The other reality is that weight loss doesn't have to be difficult. In fact, your weight loss journey can be filled with self-discovery. "A-ha" moments occur when you realize that you have made weight loss more difficult than it has to be. This leads to satisfaction and exhilaration when you finally reach your health goals ... and understand how to maintain your weight for life. Yes, it can be done!

Studies show (and I agree) that support is critical to short and long-term weight loss success. Some reasons support is critical include: goal re-affirmation and exposure to additional weight loss information and strategies. Support will provide accountability and encouragement. You need support to acknowledge your progress and to keep you going during the times you need it most. So what do I recommend? In a nutshell, find a buddy to lose weight with and enlist support from family/friends. Here are some steps to building a good weight loss support system:

1. See if there is a family member/friend/co-worker who would be seriously interested in losing weight. Buddy up with them and share your specific and realistic weight loss goals.

Work out a plan together with regards to how often you will "check-in" with each other. The buddy system works wonderfully as long as individuals are committed.

2. Enlist the support of others that can help keep you on track such as other family/friends and co-workers or professionals who provide individualized counseling, education and fitness. When determining your support system, make sure these individuals are successful themselves and committed to helping you succeed (not sabotaging your best efforts).

3. Enlist your own personal support (sounds crazy I know). You can be your best cheerleader as you learn to replace negative self-talk with positive self-talk.

As you lose weight, you will experience feelings of exhilaration and pride. However, some people may also experience fear as they move successfully towards their goal – you, your views and experiences, how others may treat you, and life in general may change somewhat as you become or feel healthier. Acknowledge that this may be the case – embrace it rather than let it sabotage your best efforts – talk to a professional so you can work through these feelings, rather than let them cause you to slip back into less healthy but more comfortable or perceived "safer" ways of life.

What can Mary Beth do? Mary Beth can follow the steps above and implement them in her life. This is obviously easier said than done and she has tried numerous times before. This is an indication that she will need professional help. The good news is that there are experienced professionals available that do this every day (and like me love it!). Having someone to support her will also be helpful since it doesn't appear as if that has been a part of her plan in the past. Remember, you are often products of your environment. Mary Beth will want to surround herself with like-minded people who want weight loss success or have already attained it ... not someone who will sabotage her efforts out of fear, jealousy or other negative reasons.

CHAPTER 8

I EXERCISE ALL OF THE TIME AND STILL DON'T LOSE WEIGHT – WHAT'S WRONG?

Meet Chuck: Chuck is frustrated to say the least. He is 38 years old and has a busy life working long days with the local cable company and keeping up with his young family. Chuck wants (and needs) to lose about 25 pounds and figured it would be easy if he just went back to the regime he had when he played football. He is working out every day combining cardio (running outside or on the treadmill) and pumping iron – even going as heavy as he can. He feels a little better but the scale hasn't budged – and he has really, really been trying. Chuck wants to continue his work-outs but needs to see the scale and his waistline go down or else he's about ready to throw in the towel!

You may wonder which is more likely to produce weight loss – diet or exercise. Many studies have compared weight-loss resulting from changing diet versus increasing activity. Overall, research has shown that dietary changes produce more weight loss than changes in exercise. However, it has also been shown that changes in one kind of behavior can lead to changes in the other, especially among women. You may be surprised to learn that initially, weight loss plans that focus on dietary change produce 2-3 times greater weight loss than those that focus on exercise. Why is this?

It appears that it is easier to cut back on calories in the foods you eat than to burn those same amount of calories through exercise. It is a fact that in general, your caloric intake far exceeds the amount of calories you could burn through typical exercise. For example, steady walking for one hour burns approximately 176 calories and one *ounce* of fat contains approximately 220 calories. That means that after one hour of steady walking you will not even have burned one ounce of fat! For most people it is a lot easier to restrict calorie intake than to burn off every-thing eaten.

Is it possible to lose weight by exercise alone? Yes it is, but, depending on what you eat, you might have to do some very serious, intense and lengthy exercise sessions to get results. You would likely find that when you exercise intensely for long durations, you won't lose any weight. In fact, you may find yourself eating more because you are hungrier and to some degree feel entitled because you are working out so hard. You also may get very tired and less likely to make good food choices and practice portion control.

Most experts (myself included) agree that although diet and exercise are both important, if you only focus on one of them, you will be much more successful if you focus on diet rather than exercise. That does not mean that I am advocating diet alone. In fact, for long-term success, a combination is recommended and usually necessary. This is because of the many health benefits that result from a combination of both diet and exercise.

It is very important to maintain or increase lean body mass as you lose weight. It can be very difficult to maintain lean body mass through diet alone. Resistance training/weight training increases your muscle and muscle burns more calories than fat – even at rest. The combination of increasing calorie expenditure through working out and decreasing calorie intake through healthy dieting will result in the reduction in weight that you seek. This is a far more effective way to drop your excess pounds!

What should Chuck do? Chuck is serious and motivated. This is great! Chuck should get a baseline body composition analysis (available free in most weight loss offices such as CFWLS). He will need to monitor his lean body mass (LBM) and fat percentage with weekly body composition analysis as he continues on his quest. Chuck is likely over-exercising which can cause injury among other things. He will need to work with an expert to establish a meal plan high in quality protein with controlled carbohydrates and get plenty of water (at least 64 ounces per day). When he combines a proper nutritional plan with a balanced cardio/resistance training work-out, he will begin to see the results he desires.

Corinne's Story

I have struggled with my weight as long as I can remember. Continual ups and downs. In July of 2012, I was in one of those up times and couldn't get my weight under control. I was heading towards a number that I never wanted to get to again. I decided that I had to do something. I had only gotten to this number just after my son was born.

The previous year I had made some significant changes in my personal life. It was all about finding ME again. It just so happens that I also found the love of my life. I finally found a partner that would support me, help me, and encourage me to go for it. His support and the support of my family and friends led me to finally realize that I can put me first. I wanted to get back into biking and participating in triathlons.

It was time to take control. I looked at some of the weight loss programs that I had done in the past and did not find that they were all that motivating this time. I had driven by Dr Clark's Weight Loss Center before and decided to check them out. The initial consultation explained all the options available which included surgical and non-surgical options. I chose the non-surgical option.

The program also included the Weight Management University (WMU). WMU provides you with supporting information and tools for your journey. You are in control of your journey and the program is there to support you.

In April of 2013, I rode 100 miles on my bike in one day for the Tour d Cure, in May I rode in the MS150, 150 miles in 2 days and on August 18, 2013, I participated in a sprint triathlon. I am still on my weight loss journey but with the support of my love, my family and friends and the tools from WMU, I know I will be successful. My goal for 2014 is the Iron Girl Triple Crown. It includes a 1/2 marathon and 2 sprint triathlons.

Before

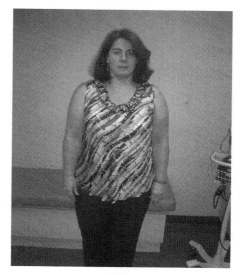

After

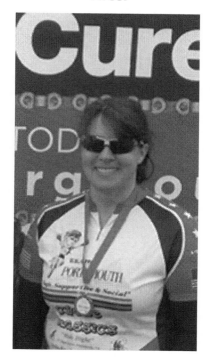

CHAPTER 9

My metabolism has tanked & my belly keeps getting bigger — why is this happening and what can I do?

*M*eet Sue: *Sue is depressed and afraid. She watched her mother and other family members (men and women) age with an ever-growing apple shape. Not only did they develop this pronounced truncal obesity, they experienced many of the diseases that come along with it such as diabetes, hypertension, back pain and sleep apnea. She is headed down the same track and desperately wants to get off this train. Sue wonders if it is possible or if her genetic predisposition has locked her into the same fate.*

Welcome to "middle age". I am not making light of this ... although the term does fit the increasing number of middle age people with expanding waists. This increased accumulation of fat around your mid-section is referred to as truncal obesity. This is caused by the accumulation of visceral fat or fat accumulating around your major organs. This visceral fat is thought of as the "least healthy" fat because it is more sensitive to insulin which increases the likelihood of added fat storage (compounding the problem). So, why do you gain weight in your abdominal area as you age? Some of the basic reasons include:

1. As you age, you have an increased likelihood of becoming carbohydrate sensitive and insulin resistant (resulting in higher circulating levels of insulin). This will be explained in more detail below, but essentially, insulin is the hormone released by the pancreas that causes you to store fat. In particular, it causes you to store fat around your internal organs (visceral fat). Visceral fat tends to be more sensitive to insulin so as insulin levels go up with age, you are more prone to fat deposits in your abdominal area. This affects both men and women.

2. As you age, you lose lean body mass. Now from previous chapters, you know that lean body mass is critical for maintaining or improving your metabolism. After the age of 28 or so, you lose about 1% of your lean body mass per year if you are not taking steps to maintain/increase it. Lean body mass helps pro-

tect you from carbohydrate sensitivity and insulin resistance. Thus, if it is decreasing, your risk for developing carbohydrate sensitivity and insulin resistance increases ... This affects both men and women.

3. As women age and reach menopause, it is harder to lose weight and easier to gain weight (this is real). Your hormones are changing. Briefly, as you age, your estradiol levels will decrease. Estradiol is a hormone made by the ovaries that helps you preserve lean body mass and is "weight stable". If these levels go down, it is easier for you to gain weight. At the same time, your production of estrone increases. Estrone is a type of estrogen that is not only made by the ovaries but also made by your fatty tissue. Estrone encourages fat storage (particularly around your middle). Thus, if you are storing more fat, you are compounding your weight problem since that additional fat causes the production of even more estrone and the cycle continues and truncal obesity worsens. This problem was also previously discussed in Chapter 5.

You may be wondering if estradiol and estrone affect men the same way. Men actually produce some estradiol but it is a very small amount. However, as they gain visceral fat, they do produce increased levels of estrone which results in the same cycle. Men are also affected by their testosterone levels (women are as well but to a much lesser degree). Testosterone is a hormone that helps to maintain lean body mass and is considered weight neutral. The production of testosterone decreases as you age. This also compounds the truncal obesity problem.

Insulin is a hormone that is extremely important to understand when it comes to weight loss. Interestingly, it is also a hormone that's production can be manipulated (especially by what you eat). This is helpful when it comes to treatment and options for successful weight loss.

I will simplify this as much as possible here. These are concepts that are extremely important to understand. Insulin is a hormone made by the pancreas and helps keep your blood sugars in a normal range. The higher your blood sugars go, the more insulin is released to help bring your sugar level back down. The fasting insulin tells you how much insulin it takes to keep your blood sugar at the fasting level. That is insulin's main job. It tries to keep blood sugars in a normal range. It does this by facilitating the transfer of sugar molecules out of your blood stream and into your cells. Subsequently, the blood sugar comes down. But this also means that the sugar content in the cells goes up. Your cells then need to "do something" with those sugar molecules.

The cells generally only have two choices of what to do with the sugar: use it immediately for energy or store it for later. Most of your cells cannot store sugar as sugar. They must convert it to fat (which it can do very efficiently). So if the cell does not need the sugar molecules for energy immediately, it stores them – as fat. So ... **insulin is a fat storage hormone.** Insulin also does some other things which are potentially detrimental to your health: increases cholesterol and triglycerides, increases blood pressure, and increases water retention.

The "drive through version" (reviewed in much more detail in the CFWLS Weight Management University™ program) is that anything you can do that will bring insulin levels down will help your overall health. When insulin levels come down and stay low, you mobilize fat ... not store it. And ... isn't that the point of a weight loss plan? So the real question you have then is – How do you stay in "fat burning mode" NOT "fat storing mode"?

Fortunately, insulin is one of the few hormones which you have some control over. Insulin only goes up when blood sugars go up – in order to bring blood sugars back down. So the way to bring insulin levels down is to keep your blood sugars as low in the normal range as possible. The lower you keep your blood sugars, the lower your insulin levels stay.

So what keeps blood sugars low? The simple version - avoiding carbohydrates (especially simple, refined carbohydrates) is what keeps blood sugars low. As I mentioned before, all carbohydrates are eventually converted to sugar molecules.

So any carbohydrate can potentially increase your blood sugar. The bottom line to all of this is that it takes a low carbohydrate diet to bring insulin levels down.

What should Sue do? Don't despair. Heredity plays a factor with regards to mid-life weight gain but Sue can positively influence her destiny and so can you. Sue needs a visit with an experienced weight loss physician, a laboratory work-up, history & physical and development of a nutrition, fitness and behavioral plan that will work for her. Sue can effectively learn how to manipulate her hormones for optimal health by the foods she eats and the inclusion of resistance training exercise.

CHAPTER 10

I'VE BEEN TOLD I AM PRE-DIABETIC.
WHAT DOES THAT MEAN?
CAN IT BE REVERSED?

Meet Tammy: Tammy is an attractive 39 year old woman who is a hard-working wife, mother and volunteer for the schools her 3 children attend and her church. Her calendar is full because she has a hard time saying "no" and genuinely loves being involved and helping others. Tammy is always on the go and has had a hard time fitting in anything that benefits her. In fact, in her mind, that might be a little bit selfish since her top priorities are her children, husband, church family and school/community causes. Tammy recently had a mandatory life insurance check-up and was told she was "Pre-Diabetic". Of course, there could be worse diagnoses, but she is extremely fearful of a life filled with blood tests, medications, needles and all of the long-term complications associated with diabetes. She has had a wake-up call and understands it is likely related to the 40 pounds she has gained since the birth of their first child ten years ago. Tammy requested an immediate appointment to see what she could do about this situation. It's time to "figure this out" and take action.

Generally people don't wake up one morning with pre-diabetes or Type II diabetes. There is a progression that may or may not be recognized or diagnosed. In fact, it is estimated that up to 80% of the diabetic Americans are insulin resistant. Sadly, most are going undiagnosed at this stage where it can fairly easily be determined and reversed. The continuum generally progresses from carbohydrate sensitivity (explained in chapter 1) to insulin resistance, then pre-diabetes and finally a Type II Diabetes diagnosis.

Remember your cells are being exposed to high levels of sugar (glucose) repeatedly, over and over, throughout the day, day after day, year after year. Eventually, the muscle cells that need to receive the glucose begin to reject or ignore the over-abundance of sugar that they are being bathed in. But your body is so determined to keep your blood glucose levels at a normal 80 to 100 that it signals the pancreas to secrete more and more insulin to do the same job it did with so much less. Your cells do what is called "down regulating".

Just as your nose "down regulates" smell. Have you ever walked into a room that had a very heavy odor, good or bad, but after a period of time the odor is less obvious to you. Your nose helped you out by "down regulating" that odor.

Your body becomes less sensitive to the insulin as it is bombarded by it repeatedly. Your pancreas will respond by secreting more and more insulin to get the job done. This in turn desensitizes your cells even more and the cycle continues.

Insulin resistance develops when your body starts ignoring what the insulin is trying to accomplish, leaving you with higher levels of circulating insulin levels, even though your blood glucose is in the normal range. Insulin levels continue to increase until your body's ability to make it wears out.

These high insulin levels may go undetected for as many as fifteen years before fasting blood sugars show in the abnormal range. Meanwhile, the elevated insulin has caused an increase in abdominal fat, hypertension, and high cholesterol readings.

Simply looking at only your fasting glucose levels does not determine how hard your pancreas is working at keeping your levels in the normal range. A *fasting insulin* level helps.

According to most lab value interpretation the normal range for insulin levels is 6-35microU/ml. This range is far too wide to be considered effective in identifying those predisposed to insulin resistance. The best fasting insulin range can be considered less than 7 microU/ml.

The diagnosis of pre-diabetes is given when you actually start seeing your fasting glucose levels increase. The blood sugar range noted most often is 100-125mg/dl. After years (sometimes between 7-15 years), the pancreas just can't keep up with the demand and requires some help. This is usually in the form of oral medications and a formal Type II (adult onset) diabetes diagnosis is made.

These medications will help, but if not diagnosed early enough one may progress from oral medication dependent diabetes to insulin dependent diabetes. This is where the pancreas has lost its ability to produce enough insulin and daily insulin injections are needed.

High Insulin levels also create other medical issues such as triggering fat storage, converting blood sugar to triglycerides and encouraging the kidneys to retain sodium (salt) thereby retaining water.

How can you reverse the effects of carbohydrate sensitivity and insulin resistance?

There are two key elements to help control and *reverse* the effects of carbohydrate sensitivity and insulin resistance: exercise and a change in your dietary intake.

Reducing your carbohydrate intake relieves the pancreas from secreting high amounts of insulin. And since insulin is a prime regulator of fat storage it would make sense to keep your insulin levels low or at least from large swings. The best way to keep your insulin levels low is to avoid eating carbohydrate foods (especially simple carbohydrates).

Another method to control your insulin levels would be to increase your lean body mass (muscle). Since your muscle mass can store carbohydrates as glycogen, the more muscle mass you have the better you will utilize the carbohydrates you do consume.

The best method to increase your lean body mass is to exercise, particularly resistance training. Exercise has an insulin like effect on lowering your blood sugars. The longer you work out or the higher the intensity of your workout, the better effect at lowering your blood sugars.

You have just read how you're eating and habits allow the progression from carbohydrate sensitivity to insulin resistance and ends as Type II diabetes. This should give you a better understanding on how to improve your weight loss and metabolically change the way your body utilizes food. Reversing these conditions takes knowledge and effort, but is possible.

What can Tammy do? Tammy can take comfort in the fact that she received her pre-diabetes diagnosis. The sooner she takes control the better. Losing even up to 10% of her body weight can begin to reverse these numbers. Tammy needs to know her numbers (Fasting Glucose, HbA1C, and insulin) and review them with her expert physician. She needs to know her effective carbohydrate levels even once she loses her excess weight and is in her maintenance phase. She should also make exercise a regular part of her daily routine. Finally, Tammy should eliminate eating three large meals and eat 3 small meals with a protein based snack (i.e. turkey/cheese) during the day. Tammy will be able to avoid sugar swings by keeping her snacks and meals balanced so the protein portion is equal to or higher than the carbohydrate level.

CHAPTER 11

WHY IS IT SO EASY TO GAIN WEIGHT AND YET SO HARD TO LOSE IT?

*M*eet Tricia: *Tricia starts a new diet nearly every Monday. Then she loses weight throughout the week when her schedule is a bit more controlled. The weekend comes and yahoo! It's time to relax and enjoy time with family and friends. When Monday comes, she starts to lose the same 2-3 pounds all over again ... never getting ahead. She wonders, why does it take so long to lose weight and yet in a matter of one or two nights, any weight lost has returned and then some!*

Have you ever questioned why it appears to be easier to gain weight than to lose it? Putting on weight doesn't seem to be a problem for most people but losing it, on the other hand, becomes a struggle. It can be very demoralizing to watch your weight increase by several pounds after one weekend of relaxed food choices, especially if your routine is altered. When you finally decide to buckle down and reduce your food intake, it seems to take much longer than a few days to see it go back down to where it was previously. Why is that?

One of the reasons you may find it easier to gain weight than to lose it is because it is so much easier to eat just an extra 200 calories a day resulting in added pounds than to subtract 200 calories each day from daily food intake. There are too many treats and temptations around that encourage you to consume more. You may not really be aware of the concentrated calories you consume when you give yourself permission to indulge a little. In addition, you may have started with just one bite of an indulgence but before you know it (especially if alcohol is involved), you have eaten the whole thing and perhaps another high carbohydrate "treat".

In today's society there are many foods that are highly concentrated in calories and it is easy to underestimate your intake. Junk food and take out restaurants have made losing weight a big challenge for anyone who can't resist temptation. Studies have found that the body burns calories more slowly than normal after weight is lost which means that you have to pay attention to lowering your caloric intake accordingly otherwise you can gain weight quickly with relative ease.

Weight loss requires more effort than weight gain. When you want to lose weight you have to work hard by paying attention to everything you put in your mouth. Gaining weight doesn't require much thought. Not worrying about it is way too easy.

Gaining weight is also a natural survival response. As the human race evolved you had to endure lengths of time with sporadic food sources. Your body was forced to become very efficient at storing and keeping fat that would be needed for energy in lean times. Subsequently, there was no hurry to lose it.

Another key factor to rapid/quick weight gain has to do with the water content in your body. Have you ever noticed how the scale drops fairly rapidly when you begin a weight loss program and then a few weeks into the program your numbers begin to move down more slowly? At this point you can become discouraged and even decide to give up all of your efforts. You may get caught up with numbers on a scale and either don't realize or overlook the fact that you are predominantly losing water weight.

The human body is about 60% water and water is lost from

the body by breathing, sweating and urination. All water losses are replaced by drinking and eating. How you balance the water coming in, to the water leaving our body differs from one individual to the next and changes in your water balance can vary considerably from one day to the next.

Here are a few things to take into consideration regarding water balance in your body. What causes your body to gain water weight?

1. *Sodium* is present in salt and causes you to retain water. You can gain up to 5 pounds overnight because of excess sodium. If you have ever eaten a meal high in salt the night before weighing the following morning – you know what I'm talking about.

2. When you eat *complex carbohydrates* your muscles stores it as glycogen and this retains three times its weight in water. That is why your scale reads higher the day after you have consumed more carbohydrates than usual.

3. There are also a few *supplements* such Creatine that can cause you to gain water weight.

4. Some medications and hormones will also increase your water retention resulting in a higher number on your scale.

What causes your body to lose water weight?

1. Decreasing your intake of sodium and/or carbohydrates. This can be done by simply reducing your overall food intake because you will automatically consume less sodium and carbohydrate by eating less.

2. All food contains some water and eating less means consuming less fluid. Taking in less fluid than your body uses will show weight loss on the scale, however, it can be dangerous if fluid is not replaced adequately. Drinking water also helps to prevent water retention.

3. If you break down muscle protein as you lose weight, you will also show water loss since the protein in your muscle holds up to 4 times its weight in fluid. You really don't want to lose muscle as you lose weight because you will diminish our ability to burn calories.

4. Water depletion through activity and/or by being out in the heat will also cause water loss and a lower number on the scale - but it is not safe. Wearing sweat suits in the gym also causes dehydration and not fat loss as so many people assume.

The bottom line is that when you begin a weight loss program your fluid balance is altered and you may see an immediate poundage loss on the scale that will slow down as your body adjusts. With approximately 3,500 calories in one pound of fat, you would have to cut back 500 calories a day to lose one pound of fat in a week. All the extra weight lost in water will return as fast as it disappeared! Checking your body fat measurements is a much more accurate way of establishing real fat loss. No fast weight loss could ever be fat loss because fat cannot be burned that quickly.

What can Tricia do? Tricia will see long-term success with consistency. Weight loss is hard work. She will do herself a favor if she is able to plan ahead. Not just for the weekdays, but for the weekend too. Journaling, taking "safe" foods with her to weekend parties, focusing on socializing instead of eating at events, trying not to deprive herself so much during the week causing her to "go crazy" on the weekend are all suggestions that work very well. It can also be very helpful for Tricia if she kept her goals or a picture of her goal/ultimate reward with her to remind herself again that "She can do it!" And "It is worth it!"

CHAPTER 12

Do I have to take vitamins and supplements to lose weight? What are the most important ones and why?

*M*eet Joe: *Joe despises taking any type of pill. He prides himself on this and refuses to take any sort of vitamin while trying to lose weight. It's just not for him!*

No matter how well you eat, vitamin supplementation is not only helpful, but recommended for nearly everyone. This is an extensive topic. You will need to talk with your expert physician regarding your particular needs. However, in the meantime, I will discuss the ones I feel are generally recommend throughout your weight loss and weight maintenance journey. These include Multivitamins, Magnesium-Potassium, B-Complex, Essential Fatty Acids, Calcium and Vitamin D.

It is also important to note that the vitamins you choose should be pharmaceutical grade (meeting the most stringent standards in the industry) and designed for ease of digestion and superior absorption. Quality does matter when it comes to vitamin supplementation.

Multivitamins: Everyone should take a good multivitamin. It is amazing to me how common vitamin deficiencies are. Remember that the RDA is the absolute minimum required to prevent deficiency diseases for most people. The RDA has nothing to do with optimum amounts for best health. Since the FDA does not oversee over-the-counter vitamins or mineral and herbal supplements, using pharmacy grade vitamins are your best bet on bioavailability of the product in question (and sometimes even if it contains what the label claims). A typical dose is usually on the bottle – usually 1-2 per day.

Magnesium-Potassium: During weight loss your body tends to waste both magnesium and potassium. Both of these minerals are essential to normal muscular and cardiovascular function. Magnesium is involved in over 300 biological reactions throughout the body. It can help prevent/treat fatigue. If you are prone to muscle cramps – you need to add this supplement. Typical doses are 1-4 tablets daily with food.

B-Complex: B-vitamins are often referred to as "energy vitamins" since they are important cofactors for many of your body's energy producing biochemical equations. They tend to make these energy producing steps run more efficiently. Vitamin B-12 is often considered the most important, but all of the B-vitamins are essential to your overall health and well-being. Activated B-vitamins are already in a form the body can use immediately and therefore – bioavailability and use is more efficient. A typical dose is 1-2 tablets per day.

Essential Fatty Acids (EFA's): Take them – they're just good for you. By taking fish oil supplements, Omega-3 fatty acids are ingested in their biologically active form. They can be directly used to support cardiovascular, brain, nervous system, and immune function. The mini-soft gels sold at CFWLS are smaller and have a natural lemon flavor to prevent a "fishy" after taste. Check to see if the EFA you are considering is ultra-filtered to guarantee removal of mercury and other possible contaminants. Most people should take 2-soft gels per day.

Calcium: You may think of calcium as essential for those young growing bones. However, it is essential for all stages of life. Yes, 99% of our calcium intake is dedicated to our bones and teeth but that additional 1% is required for cellular functions. It helps regulate muscle contraction, nerve transmission, as well as cellular permeability. Too little calcium and you set yourself up for osteoporosis, the weakening of your bones, predisposing you to fractures. But it also may be linked to rising blood pressures.

An adequate intake of calcium through the combination of foods and supplements are age dependent. Your best food sources are sardines, yogurts, cheeses and milk as well as tofu, salmon, broccoli, turnip and collard greens. Sesame seeds and almonds are also additional sources. To maximize your calcium supplement one should take no more than 500mg at a time, accompanied with Vitamin D and taken with meals.

Vitamin D is appropriately called the "Sunshine Vitamin" due to your natural ability to produce it in response to sunlight. Vitamin D is actually a hormone that your body can manufacture on its own. However, as you age, your ability to produce it declines as well as your aversion to soak up mid-day sun. In addition to your need for Vitamin D's presence to absorb calcium, more and more studies have found the importance of this vitamin for your immune system. Recent studies have also shown that those people that are overweight or those with diabetes have a higher rate of Vitamin D deficiency. Most people need to take about 2000 units per day. Having your Vitamin D levels checked is being more accepted and recommended by health care providers. You should know your Vitamin D levels.

What can Joe do? No one is going to force Joe to take vitamins. He can read about the benefits and discuss them with his expert physician and make an educated decision. Joe would do himself a favor if he took at least some of the most important ones. These are the ones that he is not likely getting in his diet and are very helpful when in a weight loss phase and beyond. These include: Multivitamin, EFA's Magnesium/Potassium Aspartate and B-Complex.

CHAPTER 13

How can I effectively handle saboteurs (situations and people) that get me off track?

Meet Maria: *Maria is extremely hard on herself. She uses the words "I can't" way too often and has a downward cast to her eyes when she speaks. She wants desperately to lose weight but comes from a large Italian family that is full of wonderful traditions. The problem is that many of them include food – and lots of it. She grew up with the proverbial "eat" from her grandmother who she adores. She doesn't want to hurt anyone's feelings but her own actions coupled with her family and events has made losing weight very difficult. As soon as she loses a little bit of weight, someone says "you are getting too thin" or "how thin do you want to get*

– you look great just as you are". Unfortunately, she is about 45 pounds overweight. Maria doesn't want to go on like this but isn't sure what to do about it.

Saboteurs can come in many forms. They are hard to handle and it takes practice and guts to overcome some of the people and situations you may face in light of any success ... especially weight loss success. You wouldn't think it would be that way but we see it frequently. Fortunately for you, there are ways to manage saboteurs quite effectively. In this chapter three different saboteurs will be addressed and more importantly – exactly how to manage them. The first is you – yes self-sabotage. The second is other people who attempt to sabotage your efforts. The third is sabotaging situations such as vacations and office parties.

Sabotage has been defined as the "act of hampering, deliberately subverting or hurting the efforts of another," or "the deliberate action to destroy property or equipment." But what is it when you try to do damage to yourself? Why on earth would you sabotage yourself? Let's examine some of the reasons.

Self–Sabotage:

Have you ever had a goal in mind but never seem to reach it? You want to achieve the goal. You have the knowledge you need to get there. You even work at achieving that goal, but it continues to be unobtainable.

Maybe it all starts with the goal you have in mind. Is it realistic? Is it attainable in the period of time you have allowed yourself? Review your personal goals using the "SMART" method. Are they Specific, Measurable, Achievable, Realistic and Time-specific? You may have all these correct but is it realistic? Losing 60 pounds in one month sets you up for immediate failure.

Doing too much too soon can easily set you up for failure. Learning a little at a time allows you to assimilate those changes slowly into your lifestyle. Are you saying you need to exercise for an hour daily when you loathe just the thought of it? You may not even make it through the first 10 minutes and the thoughts of failure start floating around in your head. That is why *small* behavioral steps are encouraged here at CFWLS. This approach is more effective for long-term change.

Many people also have the "excuse for every occasion" type of thinking. "I would have stuck with my meal plan but I had to travel last week." "I never made it to the grocery store." "I forgot to pack my lunch." "The office had a party." ...The list is endless as to why you *can't* stick with your meal plan. Stop using all that energy thinking of excuses and use that time thinking of your end result. If you focus on the finish line, rather than the process, your goals are much more achievable.

You can be your worst enemy when it comes to your sabotaging thoughts. Do you have an internal dialogue that sounds like a tug of war between something you want to do but feeling like you shouldn't? For example, you really want to exercise after work but when you get home you start thinking about all the other things you should do. Instead, change your thinking immediately to how you will feel after your workout. You'll be satisfied with yourself that you did and be glad it's completed. You will also feel happier that you are now that much closer to your goal.

Another method of self-sabotage is relying solely on your will power. Of course your will power plays an important role, but you need to help yourself by setting up a helpful environment. Cleaning out your cabinets and refrigerator of all the high risk foods and replacing them with "better choices" will lower that constant pressure to resist. Keeping your trigger foods out of sight, or better, out of your house, will go a long way in helping combat lack of willpower. Keeping your refrigerator and cabinets full of better choices helps you resist the "empty fridge … must go out to dinner syndrome". But take caution here – try not to over stock your cabinets. This too, can be a sabotaging action. Studies have shown the more food that is available in your cupboard, the more you tend to eat. Having the right amount seems to be important in your eating habits. If you must keep less desirable foods in the house for children or others, place them in a separate bag and/or plastic storage container and in an "off limits" cabinet so you have limited access.

Listening to how you feel will help you in counteracting those sabotaging thoughts. Emotional eating is counterproductive to your weight loss efforts. When you feel bored, lonely or stressed, that temporary satisfaction you feel after eating a calorie laden dessert quickly turns into "what was I thinking?" That is the question that needs to be answered. What were you thinking? Examining your thoughts prior to reaching for the Doritos may be a critical clue to your need for that sabotaging action. Journaling your thoughts during those moments may show some insight into your behavior. Once you are aware of those thoughts you can then work at changing them.

Don't do it alone. Thinking you can overcome these sabotaging thoughts without help can leave you confused and frustrated. Talking it over with a trusted friend or your counselor at CFWLS is a great first step in coming up with a plan – that is what we are here for!

Another method of self-sabotage is being inconsistent with your weight loss plan. In order to break a bad habit one must replace it with a new habit. To create a new habit you must be as consistent as possible or it will never become a new habit. Journaling is a great example of this. If you consistently journal after every meal it will become second nature and you will be able to track your carbohydrate, protein and calorie intake easily.

Combating Self-Sabotage Behavior:

1. Set realistic goals. Lose that weight slowly and purposely. Focus on the end result when exercising, not the negative thoughts.

2. Throw away the excuses. Spend your energy on ways to achieve your goals not how to get out of them.

3. Don't be in a hurry. What you want to obtain is a lifestyle change and that takes time.

4. Keep your kitchen well stocked with the foods allowed on your meal plan.

5. Try not to over buy.

6. Keep negative thinking at bay. Replace it with what you are doing right.

7. Cleaning that kitchen immediately after serving your plate may help you from going back for seconds.

8. Pre-planning your meals and activity for the day helps you stay on track.

9. Journaling your thoughts may determine if your eating is emotionally based.

10. Replace your emotional eating with another healthier activity.

11. Be consistent in your efforts.

How Others Sabotage Your Efforts:

Having a good support system to surround you while you are trying to achieve your weight loss goals is vital. They praise your efforts, notice and comment favorably on the little changes you have made. They pick up your spirits and help you get back on track when things start slipping. Wouldn't it be great if everyone you knew did this for you?

Being cognizant of those that support you and those that don't is the first step to protect yourself from saboteurs. Saboteurs can come in two varieties, the unconscious saboteur and the conscious saboteur.

The unconscious saboteurs appear to be supportive and believe they are being helpful, but they actually knock you off track by acting out of habit. Your husband may bring home a celebration cake for the 10 lbs you lost. Your friend may take you to your favorite restaurant that serves only fried foods or pasta dishes.

Both you and your husband have always celebrated achievements with food so why would this be any different? Your friend knew that this use to be your favorite restaurant. When did it change? Effectively communicating the changes that you are making is a great way to squelch those unconscious saboteurs.

The conscious saboteur may be more obvious such as the friend that says, "Just one won't hurt". Or the family member that keeps pushing her homemade baked goods at you begging you to try them. In addition to the blatant attempts to interfere with your new lifestyle, the conscious saboteurs more subtle efforts may be disrupting your workout routine by asking you to do something else when they know that is your time for fitness, or having a constant discussion with you regarding the types of foods you are now eating. You need to be aware of all types of saboteurs so you can thwart their efforts early in your journey and stay on track.

Combating Saboteurs:

1. Communicate with your friends and family assertively.

2. Have a response ready when your friend says, "Having only one won't hurt."

3. When others invite you to a restaurant that you may have been avoiding simply ask to go to another or bow out this time.

4. When others bring those trigger foods in the house have them placed out of sight.

5. When others leave their snack foods out when you asked them to be put away, have a heart to heart talk explaining you need their cooperation.

6. Stop being so polite when others insist you try their recipe. You may suggest you try it at a later date.

7. Ask for the saboteurs support. Having them work with you to obtain your goal will strengthen your friendship.

Sabotaging Events & How to Handle Them:

Yes, situations can be the culprit to sabotaging your efforts. Your home has been cleared of your trigger foods; you have started brown bagging it for lunch and minimized your dinners out – Great job!

Everything seems to be in control now. Your routine is in a nice pattern and your friends and family are on board with your changes. But what do you do with the weeklong vacation, the holiday times or the office situations that come up?

Vacations:

Vacations should be a time to enjoy and relax. Does that mean you drop all your efforts and let loose, eating everything you please and forgetting the exercise? This is where sabotaging thoughts start taking over. "I have paid for this cruise – I want to take full advantage of all the food that comes with it." "This is my vacation – I want to lie on the beach and do nothing". "I have worked hard all these months – I deserve to blow it for a week".

Changing this self-talk is the key to keeping things in check while on your vacation and planning ahead is crucial in defeating these thoughts!

What to Do:

1. Think about ways you can incorporate activity into your vacation schedule. Try a new sport.

2. Give yourself a shorter workout, but workout!

3. Check out and use the resorts exercise room. They may have a piece of equipment you have always wanted to try. They may even have group exercises available. What a great way to try out that 'yogilates' you've heard so much about.

4. Enjoy the new foods you may be exposed to if you are in a foreign country – search out different protein sources!

5. Keep your alcohol consumption in check. A drink or two might be a part of your vacation dream. However, moderation is the key.

6. The same goes for the food. Treat yourself with a splurge or two. Plan them, enjoy them, and then remember them! Get right back on track.

7. A walk on the beach is great way to relax and get some exercise ... great for those calf muscles if you are in the soft sand!

Office Life:

You have made it through your vacation and back at the office. Why is it that your office has to celebrate every event with cakes, cookies and donuts? You can smell them from your cubicle and you pass them on the way to the bathroom. The break room is a minefield of calorie-laden snacks, not to mention, everyone else's desks are topped with candies, chocolates and mints. How did this become the normal eating patterns of the everyday worker? Dealing with this on a daily basis is challenging at best.

What to Do:

1. Let your co-workers know you are trying to get healthier and lose some weight. Ask them to stop offering any special goodies they brought to the office. If you have a more relaxed atmosphere at work you may even post a little sign on your desk like they have at zoo's, 'Please don't feed the animals'.

2. If your break room is a 'minefield', start taking your break elsewhere or take a nice walk during your break. Avoiding these areas is very important in the beginning of your lifestyle change. Habits are hard to break without replacing them with new ones.

3. Your desk needs to contain lots of healthy snacks that will satisfy you when your willpower is waning. Don't forget to

bring them to that meeting where someone always places donuts on the conference table.

4. Incorporating activity to your cubicle can be a bit challenging.

5. Try being less efficient with your trips to each office you need to visit. Take the long way around or carry those folders one at a time to that meeting. It wouldn't be a bad idea to let your boss know you are trying this out … they may want to try it too.

6. Keep a stretch band or small weights at your desk to use, integrating a different exercise every hour. You could use eight different muscle groups in an eight-hour day!

The Holidays:

Studies show that approximately 53% of the American population gain weight between Thanksgiving and the New Year. There is something about the calendar during this time that says all bets are off and you can eat whatever you want. Even with the knowledge that this mentality exists and is not healthy, we are bombarded with many temptations.

There are parties. There is an increase in alcohol consumption. There can be continual socializing that is centered on rich seasonal food and drink. There are trips to the mall with free food samples and food court smells. The stress rises and the next thing you realize you have just downed that plate of chocolate cookies your next-door neighbor dropped off. Happy Holidays!

What to Do:

1. Plan for the events you will be attending. Don't go hungry. You will be less tempted to indulge in all the foods at the event if you are not starving when you arrive.

2. Plan on picking one or two special food items. Giving yourself permission to *sample* one or two foods won't set you up for feeling deprived.

3. Keep your alcohol consumption to a minimum. Drinking a glass of water with twist of lemon or lime may help.

4. Hold your drink in your dominant hand. You may be less tempted to pick at the appetizer table.

5. Keep talking to your friends away from the food area. It is hard to eat while you are talking.

6. Don't let your exercise time slip. Keep it as a priority. So what if those Christmas cards get out a little late this year. You will thank yourself on January 1 for sure!

7. This might be a good time to schedule that personal trainer. It could be that early Christmas present to you and keep you motivated through the season.

8. Find a buddy that can help you through this period. He/

she may need that accountability too.

Whether you have found your family or friends undermining your efforts at weight loss or you are letting others run your agenda, you are ultimately responsible for the changes you want to make. From sabotaging events to self-destructive thoughts, it is important for you to realize that they are all around you. You need to act on them to minimize their effects on destroying your goals and dreams.

What can Maria do? Although Maria appears to be somewhat shy, she is going to have to speak up (especially at home) if she is going to succeed. Maria needs to have her goals clearly identified along with a pre-determined weight loss plan. Then she can present her plan to her family (or at least her mother/grandmother) and sincerely ask for their support. If that is not helpful, she can involve another person who may understand or limit family time until new habits become more second nature and she experiences success. Success breeds confidence which will be extremely helpful long-term.

CHAPTER 14

WHAT'S THE BEST WAY TO OVERCOME A WEIGHT LOSS PLATEAU?

Meet Sophia: Sophia has been in the weight loss program for 2 months and has lost 15 of her desired 25 pounds. She has been beaming every time she comes into the office. Today she obtains her body composition and her face drops. She is near tears as she begins her counseling session with her weight loss coach.

Have you ever been at a point in your weight loss journey where, despite all your hard work, the scale won't budge? You haven't changed a thing but nothing seems to be happening. Chances are – you've hit a plateau! Plateaus can kill your motivation, so the first thing you need to do is to take your focus off the scale.

Your body is highly adaptive and goes through periods of adjustment. This would be a good time to concentrate on your behaviors and use alternative ways to measure your progress. Use a measuring tape or try on your favorite pair of tight jeans. If you hang in there, you will find that your inches will continue to shrink in spite of your weight staying stubbornly at the same number.

Remember that there is approximately 3,500 calories in a pound of fat, so if you continue to expend more energy than you're taking in, your weight will eventually go down. If you want to push yourself through the plateau because of pure frustration there are a few things you can do. Just remember the word CHANGE. Something needs to be changed in either your diet or exercise routine.

Let's look at your diet first:

1. Change the frequency of your meals. If you are currently eating 3 meals a day, save some of those calories for snacks in between meals and give your metabolic rate a boost.

2. Try to change what you are eating. If you are having a carbohydrate snack mid-afternoon, try replacing it with a protein one and try moving your foods around and introducing new ones.

3. Surprise your body with calorie cycling. While maintaining the same weekly calorie intake, vary it from day to day. For example, if your daily intake is 1500 calories, try having 1200 one day and 1800 the next.

What changes can you make to your exercise routine?

1. Add variety by changing your mode of exercise. If you have been walking, try adding some jogging, cycling or swimming.

2. If you aren't already strength training – now is the time to add it into your routine. Strengthening your muscles will not only strengthen your bone tissue but it will increase lean mass that will ultimately increase your metabolic rate.

3. Increase the frequency or intensity of your physical activity. Interval training, which consists of adding short bouts of higher-intensity movement into your cardio routine, is a great way to surprise your body and help to push you through a plateau.

4. Finally, workout with a friend or personal trainer. At the Center for Weight Loss Success, we have some wonderful trainers that will help to motivate you and pick up your pace.

So what other problems may be causing your plateau? We don't want to ignore anything here – you don't want to give in to frustration and slip into old habits that caused you to gain weight in the first place. You have come this far … don't stop now!

One problem may be loss of your lean body mass as you lost weight. It's a fact that muscle burns calories and losing muscle means burning fewer calories. Lean body mass uses five times the calories as fat mass so, if you lose it, your metabolism drops and your weight loss stops. So what can you do? You need to make sure you have incorporated weight training with any cardio routine. In addition, make sure you are getting adequate amounts of quality protein in (at least 80-100 grams/day).

Another problem may be your exercise plan. Your body may be getting use to your exercise choice – especially if it is the same every week. As your body gets better at performing an exercise, you can actually burn fewer calories. What do you do? Shake up your routine. Add more weight, change the intensity/duration/frequency of type of exercise. You may be a routine oriented person but try something new – it's the spice of life and you may find another activity you love!

What can Sophia do? Sophia needs to stay strong! Having a coaching appointment right after seeing this standstill on the scale is excellent. Her coach will be able to reassure her and brainstorm ways to break through the plateau and get to that final weight loss goal of 25 pounds!

CHAPTER 15

WHAT ARE CARB BLOCKERS AND ARE THEY EFFECTIVE?

*M*eet Chris: *Chris has successfully lost 60 pounds already. He is ecstatic! He has made lifestyle habits with regards to his eating and exercises 4 times a week. He has followed the program perfectly and although he has had a few plateaus, he is a success story in the making with only 15 more pounds to lose. Chris is fearful of what will happen when it is "maintenance" time. He has worked so hard, he doesn't want to fail like he has in the past. However, there are times when he is out with the guys and he wants to have a slice of pizza or a few beers and wonders about if a carb blocker would be helpful.*

Carb blockers, also called starch blockers contain an extract called phaselous vulgaris, which comes from white kidney beans. By blocking a starch-digesting enzyme called alpha-amylase, starch blockers prevent the body from absorbing carbs -- sparing you from the carb calories.[3]

Carb blockers are a natural, non-stimulant adjunctive supplement for weight loss. Many are touted to block 24-33% of carbohydrate absorption for people on low carbohydrate diets. For many of you, the amount of carbohydrate in your diet will be the single most influential factor for your weight. Carbohydrate comes in many forms, but all are eventually broken down to sugar. Therefore, the carbohydrates cause increase in blood sugars which then stimulates more insulin release (in order to control these blood sugars). But insulin also causes fat storage (i.e. weight gain). So, an important way to prevent this rise in blood sugar (and insulin) is to keep your carbohydrate intake to a minimum. Wouldn't it be nice if you didn't need to be so "strict" on your carbohydrate intake all the time?

This is where a carbohydrate blocker can provide some assistance. Typically all the carbohydrate you eat will be absorbed … except the fiber, which passes on through and tends to keep bowel function regular. Amylase is an enzyme made by your salivary glands and pancreas. Amylase helps break down complex carbohydrates (starches) into single sugar molecules which are then absorbed along the intestinal tract.

The enzyme amylase can be inhibited ("blocked") by an extract derived from white kidney beans (phaseolus vulgaris). If the amylase cannot bind with starches, then the starch cannot be absorbed. The starch will then travel down the intestine and be expelled similar to non-digestible fiber. Carbohydrate blockers can prevent the absorption of about 25%-33% of the ingested starch if taken shortly prior to a meal. In many ways, carbohydrate blockers mimic the beneficial effects of fiber with slowing absorption, decrease calorie absorption and decrease blood sugar swings.

A word of caution – some people do not tolerate large doses of fiber at one time and a carbohydrate blocker may cause some intestinal side effects such as cramps, bloating and "gas".

What can Chris do? Chris can go ahead and utilize a pharmaceutical grade carb blocker on those occasions when he is going to be having a food higher in carbohydrates. He needs to monitor himself for signs of stomach upset and not use it as an "excuse" to ingest higher amounts of carbohydrates than recommended.

[3] http://www.webmd.com/diet/features/the-truth-about-starch-blockers

CHAPTER 16

WHAT SHOULD I LOOK FOR WHEN PURCHASING WEIGHT LOSS NUTRITIONAL PRODUCTS AND VITAMINS?

*M*eet Marty: *Marty travels a lot with her pharmaceutical sales job. She is very dynamic and 48 years of age. Marty came to CFWLS 1 month ago seeking a sleeve gastrectomy weight loss surgery procedure. Even though her insurance didn't cover weight loss surgery, she has decided to move forward and is scheduled for surgery in 3 weeks. Prior to surgery, Dr. Clark recommends a "liver shrinking diet" so that patients experience weight loss prior to surgery. Even a weight loss of 10 pounds can shrink their liver* *size (since fatty liver is a common problem with people who are morbidly obese). This actually makes the surgical procedure safer and easier to perform. Marty wants to lose weight prior to surgery and wants to use supplements since it is recommended for optimal results and will be easier with her travel schedule. Marty wants to make the best choice.*

When deciding on weight loss nutritional products and vitamins, there are four main considerations:

1. Palatability: If you are going to purchase and use a nutritional product, you must like the taste. There was a time when great taste was nonexistent but that is not the case anymore. Once I verify the nutritional content, we taste test any new products and permit our patients to do the same before they buy. There are great options out there. So much so that my entire family actually chooses to have a protein shake almost every morning. It's convenient, quick and gets us off to a great start. It's more than shakes though. The sky is the limit! Whatever you purchase, make sure you like the taste or you will dread eating it, it may go to waste or you may never move on to the great tasting options available today.

2. Quality: If you choose to purchase vitamins and supplements, I recommend that you confirm that they are pharmaceutical grade rather than over-the-counter (OTC) products. I

recommend this for three main reasons:

- Pharmaceutical grade vitamins are made under conditions set forth by the American Board of Pharmacy.
- This means you can trust it for content as well as ensure the best absorption and utilization.
- OTC vitamins & minerals are not held to the same high manufacturing standards. Studies have shown that the content of the vitamin may not match what is listed on the label.

3. Weight Loss Specific: If you are seeking weight loss, then utilize the many products out there specific to weight loss. Many others have an extremely high carbohydrate content, lower protein content and are made from lower quality proteins.

4. Cost: Cost is definitely important but as a caution – sometimes you get what you pay for. More satisfying proteins such as casein are less abundant and will cost you a little bit more. Try to compare the supplement cost to the cost of a meal. It may surprise you.

As you likely know, meal replacements play an important role in weight loss for many people but are you aware that studies show that individuals who use meal replacements are much more successful in both weight loss and long-term weight maintenance. You may be wondering ... What do we consider meal replacements? Meal replacements essentially include bars, beverages and entrees.

Research shows that 74% of individuals using meal replacements with at least one meal of regular food lost and maintained 5% of their initial body weight compared to 33% of those on a reduced calorie diet with their own selected foods. That is a considerable difference.

It appears that there are several reasons why meal replacements are so effective in weight loss and maintenance. They are portion-controlled which gives individuals visual re-education. The calories are calculated correctly. Food decisions are simplified. They are convenient and easily accessible. They are already prepared. They contain improved nutrition and with a variety of flavors offered ... they also taste good.

The cost of meal replacements also makes them a good choice. In a recent study, dieters who used meal replacements actually reduced their overall food costs from baseline. The USDA found that the average American spends *at least* $100 weekly on regular food. When compared with quality meal replacements/supplements the cost of regular food often exceeds the cost of nutritional supplements.

Improvements associated with meal replacements include improved fasting glucose, total cholesterol, LDL cholesterol, blood pressure, triglycerides and insulin.

Evidence is strong that substituting at least 1-2 meals and/

or snacks daily with meal replacements is a great strategy for successful weight loss and maintenance especially for those of you have difficulty with portion control.

What should Marty do? Mary is smart to complete her liver shrinking diet. This diet can be accomplished with a variety of products. She needs to visit the CFWLS store, taste what she is interested in and make an educated purchase that she will enjoy!

Beth's Story

Losing weight has always been hard for me but Weight Management University™ has made it so much easier.

I started with a 2 week Jumpstart plan and then began WMU. The educational chapters, along with Dr. Clark's explanations on how my body responds to different foods has opened my eyes to a new way of looking at my food choices.

My counseling visits helped hold me accountable and assisted me in changing a few habits. I truly thought it was going to be difficult to stick with it and it has been completely the opposite.

Dr. Clark and his staff are very supportive and encouraging. The nutritional information and other weight loss tips offered to you is unbelievable. The fitness classes and challenges keep it fun and the other members are so supportive of each other. This was not a "diet" but a lifestyle change for me. Everything about the Center for Weight Loss Success has been a great experience!

Before

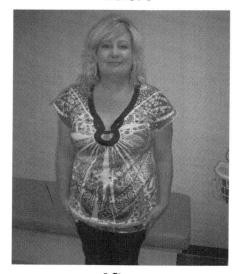

After

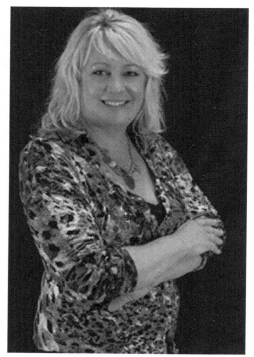

CHAPTER 17

WHAT DOES SLEEP HAVE TO DO WITH WEIGHT LOSS?

Meet Kathy: Kathy is a real estate agent. She is 55 years old and has found it difficult to sleep for a variety of reasons. Kathy is stressed about the economy and caring for her aging mother. In addition, her husband often snores and likes to fall asleep with the TV on in their bedroom.

Sleep – it's so good for you. As a routine part of counseling, we review the average number of hours you sleep each night. That is because getting enough sleep is a very important part of your weight loss plan. Lack of sleep affects your body in several ways:

1. Lack of sleep is a stressor. Stress raises your cortisol level, which in turn sends a message to your body to store fat. This hormone also interferes with your melatonin levels which is the hormone that helps put you to sleep.

2. Little or no deep, restful sleep prevents the body from building up a reserve of serotonin. Lack of adequate levels of serotonin can set you up for cravings and over-eating. This is the same hormone that is associated with depression.

3. The absence of deep restful, restorative sleep is associated with a decrease in production of growth hormone. This is the hormone that helps keep you young and fit!

Who would think so much was going on while you sleep? An occasional fretful night may not have these effects on your weight loss but continuous nights of 5-6 hours or less of sleep could be sabotaging your weight loss efforts. If you find that this is a problem for you, it needs to be addressed. Below are some tips to help you get your sleep pattern on track. If the problem persists, you need to talk to your physician expert.

1. Try to go to bed and wake up at the same time (building routine).

2. Avoid stimulants such as caffeine, nicotine or alcohol at least 2-3 hours before bedtime.

3. Make sure your room is dark.

4. Try not to watch TV, listen to the radio or read in bed.

5. Exercise is not only good for overall health but for sleep as well so don't forget to work in a work-out. As a caution you should avoid working out within 2-4 hours prior to going to bed since it usually takes a couple of hours following exercise before you are able to relax enough for sleep.

Life can be so stressful … work, bills, caring for kids/parents, laundry, cleaning, "what's for dinner?", unrealistic expectations … it goes on and on. Most feel pushed to the limit. Stress also negatively impacts sleep and weight loss.

If you are stressed (and who isn't), here are some great ways to cope and get a grip on your life and your health. Remember – if you don't take care of yourself, you can't effectively take care of others.

1. Get Active: Physical activity is one of the most important things you can do to keep stress away by clearing your head and lifting your spirits. It increases your endorphin levels, the "feel-good" chemicals in your body that leave you with a natural happy feeling. Walk, play tennis, swim, bike … find something you enjoy that will get you moving!

2. Eat Regularly: Don't forget to eat breakfast. You need that energy to tackle the day and rev up your metabolism. Make sure that you eat regular meals and fuel up with healthy foods. For that extra boost of energy grab a protein shake, some string cheese, or a protein bar.

3. Laugh: Lots of laughing can make you feel good, so watch a funny movie, some cartoons or read a joke book. Some say that laughter is the best medicine ... so lighten up and have some fun. Have fun with friends. Friends can often help you to work through your problems and let you see the brighter side.

4. Don't Go It Alone: Instead of keeping your feelings bottled up inside, talk to a friend, family member or someone in your religious community. Someone you trust or respect can help you figure things out.

5. Take Time to Relax: Stress can make us feel really tight, so it is important to find time to relax by doing such things as daydreaming, reading or listening to music. Take some relaxing deep breaths.

6. Get Enough Sleep: Getting the right amount of sleep is especially important if you are under stress. When you're tired a problem can appear to be much bigger than it really is.

7. Keep a Diary: Writing things down can get them off your chest. So, write down your feelings and events that occur.

8. Plan: Organizing your life can prevent you from becoming overwhelmed and forgetful.

9. Learn Ways to Deal with Anger: It is important to deal with anger in a healthy way so that you don't increase your stress level. Try to calm down before doing or saying anything. Tell the person you're upset with how you feel. Try to think of

ANSWERS TO THE TOP 21 WEIGHT LOSS QUESTIONS

some solutions and put them into action.

What can Kathy do? *Kathy is going to have to implement some of the stress strategies mentioned above in order to improve her sleep patterns. She is also going to have to talk to her husband about turning the TV off at night. If his snoring continues, she may want to have him evaluated for sleep apnea or make other sleeping arrangements. She should also talk to her experienced physician regarding any supplements that can help her get a good night sleep such as melatonin.*

CHAPTER 18

WILL MY INSURANCE COVER MEDICAL WEIGHT LOSS?

Meet Jean: Jean works at a local law firm as an administrative assistant. She wants to lose about 35 pounds and is interested in medical weight loss. Jean wonders if this non-surgical program would be covered by her insurance company.

This is a great question and there are a few considerations to be made prior to providing an answer. These include:

1. In what state the services are provided.

2. Whether or not the practitioner is a provider with your particular insurance company.

3. What co-morbidities (health problems) you have along

with your BMI.

In many states, medical weight loss is not a covered benefit. A common exception where nutritional counseling may be a covered benefit is if it is provided as a part of a diabetes educational program.

Since this is the case, many practitioners (myself included) actually structure their program so that for the various visits (physician, counselor, classes and personal training), the overall cost ends up being less than the cost of a typical co-pay and fees can be spread out over a period of time to make them affordable.

What can Jean do? Jean will have to verify specifics for her state/situation and then determine what is right for her. She should verify outcomes commonly attained. Depending upon her health problems, the ultimate medication, cost of missed work and physician visit savings often outweigh the cost of the program.

Elizabeth's Story

Late January, 2012, I called the Center for Weight Loss Success to make an appointment as I contemplated weight loss surgery with Dr. Clark – specifically, the sleeve gastrectomy. My husband and I went to an informational meeting to see what it was all about. At this point, I was desperate and needed help.

I have tried just about every program and product out there. I even tried starving myself and each time I actually gained weight! Finally, I asked about weight loss surgery at a local hospital and they gave me Dr. Clark's name. "God Bless" them!

However, after the seminar, I found that I actually wasn't eligible at the time for weight loss surgery. Our policy required 12 months of medically supervised weight loss and my BMI also might not have been high enough. Oh my! I cried and cried. I went to pieces because I had already tried everything and COULD NOT LOSE WEIGHT. What was I going to do? I felt even more frustrated and defeated.

After talking to Dr. Clark's office manager (such a wonderful help), she suggested I try his medical weight loss program. I could try it and if it didn't work, I could pursue surgery in 1 year. After she and my husband finally calmed me down, I agreed. What did I have to lose ... right ... exactly ... lose!! And believe it or not – THAT'S WHAT I DID – I WAS FINALLY ABLE TO LOSE WEIGHT!!!

I weighed 211 pounds when I walked in the door of CFWLS initially. I now weigh 141 pounds – Yes! I lost 70 pounds!!! I am totally amazed. You see, what I haven't told you is that I am handicapped and walk with a cane. I tried to exercise but with my disability, I am very limited in what I can do. I tire easily so exercise was not really feasible.

I don't know what your situation is but I want you to know that if I lost weight, anyone can. Know that there is hope. I know how you feel. If it wasn't for the Center for Weight Loss Success, Dr. Clark and his wonderful staff, I would not be where I am to-day ... 70 POUNDS LIGHTER!!

I am also extremely grateful for my wonderful husband and his unending love and support.

Before

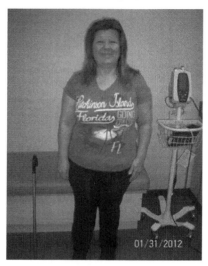

After

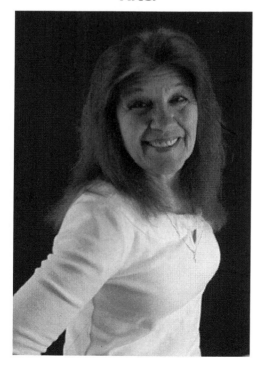

CHAPTER 19

WHAT'S THE BEST KIND OF PROTEIN? HOW MUCH DO I NEED?

*M*eet David: *David is an engineer who likes to know the analysis behind recommendations. He is savvy in that he has already researched the programs available in his area and the recommendations of each. He has chosen a program that recommends adequate amounts of protein with controlled carbohydrate intake. His goal is to lose 60 pounds within 9 months. He wants to do everything correctly and "by the book". He has some questions about protein sources and supplements and is seeking someone to clarify what is best.*

The word protein is derived from the Greek word proteios, meaning "of the first quality". Protein is essential for life (i.e. we CANNOT survive without it!!!) because it contains sulfur and nitrogen, two vital elements for every cell in your body. Protein also helps produce enzymes and hormones, maintain fluid balance, and regulate numerous vital functions, from building antibodies to building muscle. The body maintains roughly 50,000 different protein containing compounds, forming the building blocks of muscle, bone, cartilage, skin, hair and blood.

As far at your diet is concerned, there are numerous kinds of proteins, each with their own set of advantages. The right kinds can make all the difference, especially if you are trying to lose weight and build muscle. Some of the best protein comes from food. Meat has about 7 grams of protein/oz, large eggs about 7 grams of protein, and milk about 8 grams of protein/8oz. In a weight loss plan, you have to watch all the extra calories (fat, carbs) that come with food sources of protein.

1. Whey Protein: Whey protein is derived from milk (remember Little Miss Muffet and her curds and whey?). Many whey protein supplements have had most of the excess fat, cholesterol and lactose removed. Whey proteins are the most commonly used and most popular protein used in sports nutrition. They are the highest quality protein available with an excellent balance of essential amino acids.

Whey proteins are <u>very efficiently</u> absorbed and this is extremely important but this is also a potential problem. Because whey protein is so efficiently absorbed (i.e. absorbed quickly) it tends to not keep you feeling full or satisfied for any extended period of time. For this reason, it also tends to work better if used in small doses (10-20 gms) taken multiple times throughout the day. Your hunger can potentially return faster with whey protein than with other proteins.

2. Casein Protein: Casein protein is also derived from milk (the curds part of curds and whey) and is essentially whey's counterpart. It also is a very high quality protein with all the essential amino acids. While whey is absorbed very rapidly, casein forms a <u>slow digesting</u> gel in your stomach. This in turn promotes a feeling of fullness that can stave off hunger for longer periods of time. This steady stream of amino acids helps to protect against muscle breakdown.

3. Egg Proteins: Egg proteins digest at a moderate pace. Eggs are an excellent protein source and mimic the amino acid profile of muscle quite nicely. Unfortunately, eggs do have a relatively high amount of cholesterol and also arachodonic acid (mainly in the yolks). Some people are very sensitive to arachodonic acid worsening inflammatory processes. Egg proteins in supplement form (usually as albumin) have had most of the cholesterol and arachodonic acid removed.

4. Soy Protein: Soy protein is also digested at a moderate pace. Soy protein contains all of the essential amino acids, but since soy is a plant, it tends to not have quite as good of a ratio of essential amino acids as dairy or egg based protein. Therefore, it does not tend to protect muscle mass quite as well. It can still be a good alternative for those who do not tolerate dairy based proteins.

How Much Protein Do I Need?

During weight loss you need to protect (or improve) your muscle mass. A good way to estimate how much protein you require per day during a weight loss plan is to look at your body composition. Take the total number of pounds of LBM and divide by 2. Then multiply the result by 1.5. This is the <u>minimum</u> amount you will require. It is typically at least 90-100 grams/day. Again, this is a minimum. If you take in less than that you will likely be breaking down a lot of Lean Body Mass/muscle. You'll still be losing weight but you will also be losing muscle mass. The major problem long-term is that your metabolism will slow down significantly. Subsequently you will likely not lose as much weight and it will be <u>harder</u> to keep the weight off.

As far as timing goes, ideally you should use smaller doses of protein multiple times throughout the day. Starting the day off with a good dose is always a good idea (i.e. that protein shake in the morning). An example would be 20-30 grams at breakfast, 20-30 grams at lunch and 20-30 grams at dinner. Then add two 10-20 gram snacks, appropriately spaced between meals. Positioning a protein snack prior to and immediately after strenuous exercise works extremely well to build/preserve muscle mass.

High Protein Vs Adequate Protein Diets:

People often confuse what we recommend as a "high" protein diet. What I really recommend is <u>adequate</u> protein. Adequate protein is the amount of protein required to prevent loss of LBM during a weight loss plan. This is usually around 1.5x the amount needed during weight maintenance.

High protein diets are those diets that recommend taking in a much higher amount per day (2.5-4x the amount needed for weight maintenance or 400- 500 grams/day). Body builders and some professional athletes may do this. But there is <u>some sense</u> to high protein diets to help with weight loss for a few reasons. First, protein tends to be very satisfying – meaning you tend to stay "fuller" (satisfied) for a longer period of time after eating protein. Second, protein is harder for your body to digest and since digestion is "work" that your body must perform, it also then burns more calories (referred to scientifically as thermogenesis). Finally (and probably most importantly), protein tends to increase the production of the hormone glucagon as well as growth hormone. Both of these hormones tend to help you mobilize and utilize fat – that is, they <u>increase</u> weight loss!

Here's some very important information regarding protein. Some you may already know and some may really surprise you:

1. Protein is the most important macronutrient. We can't survive without protein.

2. Did you know that we have what are known as "essential" fats and "essential" amino acids in protein but nowhere is it stated that we have "essential" carbohydrates? Actually studies show that the lower limit of dietary carbohydrate compatible with life is apparently zero. Carbohydrates are the least important macronutrient.

3. The average American consumes between 76 and 100 grams of protein daily which is about 15% of your calories. As the acceptable macronutrient distribution is 10%-35%, it means that we don't eat too much protein.

4. Protein intake is an absolute requirement and is based on what stimulates protein synthesis in our body. Protein synthesis is affected by the **amount, quality** and **timing** of protein intake.

5. **So about how much do we need?** 20-30 grams of pro-

tein is needed to stimulate protein production.

6. Which protein sources are the best? Complete proteins with all the essential amino acids are best and these would include meat, poultry, fish, eggs, cheese, milk and yogurt. Combining incomplete plant protein sources such as grains with legumes or legumes with seeds is also acceptable.

7. When is the best time to consume protein? 20-30 grams of protein should be consumed at each meal. The most important time to eat protein is at breakfast because your body is "breaking down" proteins after an overnight fast. Your body does not store "extra" protein.

Here are some protein myths you should be aware of as well:

1. Protein does not cause osteoporosis. Poor protein status leads to bone loss and adult women who are most at risk for bone loss, may have the most compromised protein status.

2. Protein does not cause kidney disease. A low animal protein diet conducted over a period of 4-5 years did not cause a reduction in the incidence of kidney stones.

3. Protein does not cause heart disease. The Nurses' Health Study showed an inverse relationship between protein intake and the risk of cardiovascular disease. Obesity is the risk for heart disease and replacing dietary carbohydrate with protein improves weight loss.

What should David do? David has the information he needs to choose wisely with regards to optimal protein choices whether it is from regular food choices or protein supplements. He should continue to ask questions as he progresses through his weight loss program to make sure his protein requirement adjustments are made as necessary and he is able to stay within his set budget. He will also want to get some great recipes so that he has variety to prevent boredom of choices. He is on his way! Good luck!

CHAPTER 20

WHAT'S A BARIATRICIAN AND WHY SHOULD I CARE?

Meet Tracy: Tracy is confused. She wants to lose weight ... period. She just found out she has diabetes and she feels terrible. Tracy is scared. She did an internet search and talked to her primary care physician about what to do. She is supposed to visit a bariatrician but she isn't exactly sure what that really means.

What do all of those titles really mean? Better yet, are they important? Well, they can actually mean something significant as a part of a bigger picture. This is especially important when you choose the person(s) you are going to trust with your overall health, weight loss efforts, goals and dreams.

According to the Obesity Action Coalition[4], a bariatric physician is a doctor who specializes in helping patients lose weight without surgical intervention. Bariatricians treat obesity and related disorders. Such physicians are typically a member of the American Society of Bariatric Physicians (ASBP). Many of these physicians have obtained advanced training and certification in weight loss medicine. Board certification is determined by The American Board of Obesity Medicine (ABOM) and helps to assure quality weight loss.

Who (if anyone) you choose to help you with your weight loss journey is your decision. What's most important is YOUR outcome … YOUR results. Thus, anyone who helps you successfully meet or exceed your weight loss goal(s) is the right choice.

I value education. I value experience. I value cost-effectiveness. However, when the three come together, that's even better. As you know by now, I am a firm believer in education and then applying what you have learned. Years ago, I chose to become board certified in surgery and bariatric medicine. I also chose to specialize exclusively in the field of weight loss (surgical and medical). I do this because I love helping others. I love helping you lose weight, improve your health problems, decrease or eliminate your unwanted medications and live day-to-day life at your peak performance. Not a day in the office goes by when we don't well up with tears hearing success stories … and that's a pretty awesome day! Not only your big success stories with regards to total pounds lost but the little things…

- Crossing your legs
- Tying your shoes
- Playing on the ground with your kids/grandkids
- Becoming a firefighter again
- Getting rid of your cane and/or wheelchair
- Sitting comfortably in your car, an airplane or a ride at your favorite amusement park
- Eating a smaller amount and actually feeling satisfied
- Being a great example of healthy living for your loved ones
- Running a 5K
- Running a marathon
- Feeling confident about your body
- Playing a winning game of golf
- Exercising regularly (and enjoying it without fear of fail ure or giggles from others)
- Lowering your medication bill (or eliminating it alto gether)
- Going to fewer doctor appointments
- And so much more…

The bottom line is that you need to determine what is right

for you. In addition to the information presented in Chapter 3, utilize some questions set forth by the Obesity Action Coalition4 when selecting your bariatrician. They recommend that before you meet with a bariatrician for the first time, ask the following questions so you can feel more comfortable with their level of training and expertise:

1. Do you specialize in bariatrics?

2. Is your education in this area current?

3. What kind of initial patient work-up do you perform?

4. What is your policy on the frequency of follow-up visits?

5. If you prescribe medications, what potential side effects can I expect?

6. Do you prescribe low calorie and very low calorie diets with supplements? If so, have you received special training in monitoring patients on these diets?

You need to be ready, you need to be involved and you need to feel comfortable with your choice. Not only with the physician, but with his/her entire staff, facility, products/program, education, on-site and online support and overall "feel" you have about each of these aspects. Weight loss isn't a short-term, passing activity. Weight loss doesn't have to be hard. You need to see results. You need to feel motivated. You need to "change". However, this "change" needs to be something you can (and will) do for life. This is not a dream – what you do today deter-mines your tomorrow. You can do it!

What should Tracy do? Tracy should talk to her primary care physician regarding his/her recommendations. She can also locate a bariatrician in her area by visiting the ASBP's website at www. asbp.org and click "Locate a Physician". She can also search the internet for additional resources. At CFWLS, we offer free weekly podcasts, blog articles regarding the latest weight loss information and recipes. Tracy can visit www.cfwls.com to access these many free resources.

[4] http://www.obesityaction.org

CHAPTER 21

WHAT CAN I DO RIGHT NOW TO START LOSING WEIGHT?

Your summary action guide to success!

*M**eet YOU: You have struggled, you want and deserve success. You are special and you can accomplish whatever you set your mind to do. Your future is in your hands and you can do this!*

How often have you thought, "Tomorrow is the day, I will make my weight a priority?" Unfortunately, without the right tools, the success rate is less than 24%. It's a new day. It's a new beginning. Take that refreshing energy and go for it! Here is a tried and true 12 step plan that will help you make your personal weight loss success story a reality.

1. Get Over It – I don't mean to sound harsh, but in order to really be successful, you need to get over a few things:

- Get over thinking you are being selfish if you decide to invest in yourself and improve your eating and fitness habits (your family and the rest of the world will adjust and in time, hopefully join your new way of living).

- Get over thinking that there is a magic pill or fad diet that will work. Your habits didn't occur overnight and making true healthy changes in your life will take time and effort. I promise that your efforts will pay off exponentially and you can have fun along the way.

- Get over thinking that just what you eat or just exercise is important. Ultimate weight loss success happens when you incorporate both into your life. Successful baby steps create motivation and the drive to continue until you experience long-term positive results.

2. Make a Decision – You control your destiny. When you look at your accomplishments in life, they are usually the result of a decision you made along with your commitment to make it happen. Weight loss is no different. You will be most successful if you clearly decide what your realistic goals are (short and long-term), document them, review them every day, share them with others and monitor your progress along the way.

3. Picture This – Picture yourself at the finish line feeling your best, looking your best and showing off your newfound way of life and optimized health. The energy, the positive outlook and the vitality that goes along with weight loss and a job well done is now yours. This is the new you. This is YOUR accomplishment and will help keep you motivated as you experience expected plateau's and challenges along the way.

4. Plan, Plan & then Plan Some More – There are many choices out there with regards to weight loss and fitness. The important thing is to select a program that you can live with long-term ... not a 'diet' that works only short-term. You will need to plan your meals, schedule your activity and stick to it as if your life depends upon it ... and for many, it does. Keeping a food journal (yes, I said it) will double your likelihood of being successful. This is very important during your weight loss phase. Being "too busy" will get you nowhere fast. If you make weight loss and healthy living a priority in your life, it will get done.

5. Don't Make It Difficult – Weight loss doesn't have to be difficult. If it is, you will not likely be compliant. Whatever you do, you need to be able to admit that this is something you can do for life. Otherwise, you may be successful short-term but never truly integrate healthy habits into your life for long-term success. Your objective should be to lose fat (not your lean body mass) by controlling your production of insulin (which causes you to store fat), mobilize your fat stores and build muscle along the way by ingesting adequate amounts of quality protein and incorporating resistance training to your routine. As you age, your hormone levels may need to be evaluated and optimized along the way as well. Preserving your lean body mass (muscle) will preserve and/or improve your metabolism so that yo-yo dieting is a thing of the past. It doesn't have to be tricky. The simpler the better!

6. Get a Pal – It's no secret that people who want to lose weight are much more likely to be successful if they have adequate support. When determining your support system, make sure these individuals are successful themselves and committed to helping you succeed (not sabotaging your best efforts). Studies show (and I agree) that support is critical to short and long-term weight loss success. Some very good reasons include goal re-affirmation, exposure to additional weight loss information/strategies, accountability and encouragement to acknowledge your progress and keep going at times when you need it the most.

7. Go Slow – As you better understand your relationship with food, you will analyze your food choices and begin to 'eat to live' not 'live to eat'. You will want to slow down your eating so you can savor your delicious choices, enhance your satiety, and listen to your body's signs of true hunger and feeling full prior to feeling stuffed. In this fast paced world, going slow can be a welcomed change and actually enhance your family relationships around the table as well.

8. Eat Enough – Going through life feeling deprived is no way to live. If you aren't eating enough (and the right types of foods) you will not have enough energy to do everything you want to do, your metabolism will slow and you will likely be unhappy. You will essentially set yourself up for failure. Eating 3 meals with 2 protein snacks is ideal. Staying hydrated with water and low or no calorie beverages is also important. Getting about 30 grams of protein in at breakfast (and all of your meals) will help you feel satisfied and help maintain your lean body mass. Approximately 2/3 of the American population are carbohydrate sensitive and may also be insulin resistant so controlling your carbohydrate intake will help you avoid those nasty blood sugar rebound symptoms (lethargy, shaky, headache and feeling blah or nauseous).

9. Work in a Work-Out – Yes, it is important. No, it doesn't have to be for long periods of time. Yes, it should be something you enjoy. No, fitness 1-2 times a week is not adequate. Yes, resistance training is key along with cardio work-outs and … Yes, you can do it! Just get moving. If nothing else, wear your pedometer and gradually work up to the recommended 10,000 steps a day. Getting started with a certified personal trainer is a great way to begin. Variety is the spice of life and keeps you from getting bored.

10. Get Your Zzzzz's - Studies show that you need about 7 hours of sleep each night. Inadequate sleep has been shown to interfere with metabolism of carbohydrates and as a result, cause high blood glucose levels which increases insulin levels and results in fat storage (not good). It has also been shown to decrease leptin levels which affects your appetite (causes you to crave carbohydrates). Another significant effect is reduction in your levels of growth hormone which can result in storage of fat as well. None of this is good news. Sleep is more important than you think!

11. Talk to Yourself – Your 'self-talk' can mean the difference between success and failure. You know what I mean … it's that angel on one shoulder reminding you of your goals and how great you are doing and the devil on the other shoulder saying 'just this one won't hurt'. You have control over these situations even if you need to talk to yourself out loud or have goal reminder messages as your screen saver, in your wallet or all over your house/office. This will get easier over time as your new habits evolve and become a way of everyday life. Talk yourself through those difficult times, distract yourself or call your pal for some positive reinforcement. You are worth it!

12. Celebrate – As you progress through your journey, celebrate you and all of your accomplishments. A new outfit, pair of shoes or that gadget you've been wanting … a new piece of fitness equipment, a series with a personal trainer, a protein supplement indulgence (yes, they are really delicious) … a bubble bath, a pedicure or a new haircut. You have earned it. Isn't life grand?

What should YOU do? You should celebrate you and take steps to live the life you dream about. It is possible and it is in your hands. Follow the advice in this book and know that you are not alone. If you need help, take advantage of the resources offered here and let us know of your successful progress at *success@cfwls.com* Cheers to YOU!

Added Bonus – Dr. Clark's 7 Top Weight Loss Mistakes

1. Thinking exercise or diet alone will get you the results you want.

2. Attempting weight loss efforts for anyone other than you.

3. Going for 'low fat' instead of 'controlled carbohydrate.

4. Not monitoring your lean body mass as you lose weight resulting in loss of muscle and slower metabolism.

5. Not eating enough – feeling deprived generally results in

a rebound 'binge' and slower metabolism.

6. Having an 'all or nothing' attitude – life is meant to be enjoyed – if you make a mistake, just get back on track with the next meal … not the next week or month.

7. Weekend think ("It's the weekend so…") – plan your weekends so that they don't derail your efforts accomplished throughout the week.

Added Bonus – 30 Tried & True Weight Loss Tips You Can Begin TODAY!

These tips are tried and true. They come from Dr. Clark and the entire team at CFWLS and our successful patients! Remember, reading is one thing – applying what you learn is where you can make the most progress.

1. Start your day with approximately 30 grams of protein.

2. Stay away from foods that contain sugar.

3. Explore different tastes with a variety of spices – without adding carbs!

4. Carry a carb gram counter and your journal with you so you can analyze what may be causing your cravings or hunger.

5. Hit a plateau? Try reducing your carb intake by 5-10 grams.

6. Learn how to read food labels to count effective carbs.

7. Avoid excessive caffeine which may trigger hunger or

food cravings.

8. Eat slowly; extending the time it takes for your brain to realize you have eaten.

9. Only eat until you are satisfied, not until you are full.

10. Use smaller plates at meal times. It may help you feel like you're eating more.

11. You can have a bite of something without eating a complete piece.

12. If you have gone over your limit at a meal, forgive yourself and re-focus at the next meal.

13. Eat your meals at a table, concentrating on your food, avoiding watching TV or reading.

14. Don't use a business trip or vacation as an excuse not to follow your plan.

15. Don't miss a meal. Your body is counting on you to provide for it.

16. Always carry some emergency food with you (protein bars or nuts are good choices).

17. When eating out, engage your server in your eating plan. They may have some suggestions.

18. When eating out, ask about the ingredients of each dish.

19. Drink an 8 oz. glass of water prior to each meal.

20. Include your hunger scale in your food diary so you can

analyze any patterns and improve planning strategies.

21. Place any tempting foods in an out of the way place in your home so you don't visualize it every time you open the pantry.

22. Keep your grocery trip on a list to minimize spontaneous buying.

23. Stay to the perimeter for the grocery store. Most processed foods and higher carb foods are in the aisles.

24. Plan your day ahead of time. Then stay on track.

25. Surround yourself with supporting friends and family.

26. Return to your food diary for successful weight loss weeks and repeat them.

27. Keep your protein levels equal to or higher than your carb level with each snack.

28. Avoid carbs prior to bedtime to keep your glucose levels even throughout the night.

29. Find ways to reward yourself in ways other than food.

30. Eat to live, don't live to eat.

Added Bonus – 21 Free Videos at

www.weightlosssuccess4me.com

Index

[1] http://www.cdc.gov/obesity/data/adult.html

[2] http://www.nhlbi.nih.gov/guidelines/obesity/ob_gdlns.htm

[3] http://www.webmd.com/diet/features/the-truth-about-starch-blockers

[4] http://www.obesityaction.org

Made in the USA
Columbia, SC
25 January 2025